NATURAL PET CURES

Dog & Cat Care the Natural Way

Dr. John Heinerman

PRENTICE HALL

Library of Congress Cataloging-in-Publication Data

Heinerman, John.
    Natural pet cures : Dog & cat care the natural way / by John Heinerman.
       p. cm.
    Includes index.
    ISBN 0-13-25484-0 (ppc)   ISBN 0-7352-0036-X (p)
    1. Alternative veterinary medicine. 2. Dogs—Diseases—Alternative treatment.
  3. Cats—Diseases—Alternative treatment. 4. Herbs—Therapeutic use. 5. Herbals.
  I. Title.
  SF745.5.H45   1998
  636.089'55—dc21   98-18803
                                                  CIP

Acquisitions Editor: *Doug Corcoran*
Production Editor: *Jacqueline Roulette*
Formatting/Interior Design: *Robyn Beckerman*

© *1998 by Prentice Hall, Inc.*

All rights reserved. No part of this book may be reproduced in any form or by any means, without permission in writing from the publisher.

Printed in the United States of America

10 9 8 7

This book is a reference work based on research by the author. The opinions expressed herein are not necessarily those of or endorsed by the publisher. The directions stated in this book are in no way to be considered as a substitute for consultation with a duly licensed veterinarian.

ISBN 0-13-258484-0

PRENTICE HALL
Paramus, NJ 07652

On the World Wide Web at http://www.phdirect.com

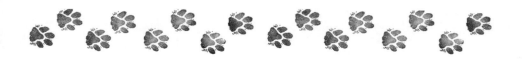

Dedicated To

The children and grandchildren of Reverend Peter J. Hofer (1919–1993) and Susanna J. Hofer (1922–1987).

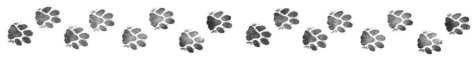

FOREWORD

In the early 1970s as a young, energetic, traditional veterinarian, on the cusp of transition toward holistic medicine, I found myself hungrily searching for any "proof" that the alternative approach had any merit at all! The veterinary literature, while replete with traditional symptom-oriented allopathic drug therapies, was virtually empty when it came to holistic health care for animals. There was a handful of veterinarians dabbling with natural remedies in their day-to-day practice. Reference materials were scarce and most therapies were extrapolated from the human alternative areas of chiropractic, naturopathic, and osteopathic approaches to human ailments.

My own personal alternative veterinary library consisted of several classical books on home remedies and folk medicine stories compiled and written by animal-loving people who rejected the medical approach, in favor of the more natural approaches of feeding whole foods, vitamins, minerals, homeopathic, and medicinal herbs. One of my primary references at this time was a small, faded green paperback book entitled *Healing Animals with Herbs* by John Heinerman, published in 1983. This little book was one of my initial entries into the use of herbs in the treatment and healing of animals.

Now, 15 years later, I find it uncanny that I have been asked to write the foreword to John Heinerman's newest book on animal health entitled Natural Pet Cures—Dog & Cat Care the Natural Way. This all seems quite apropos since I utilized John's initial book as a reference, supporting my own transition into holistic veterinary medicine.

Since the early 70's things have certainly changed with regards to the natural approach to the healing of animals. Holistic Veterinary Medicine is essentially "mainstream" with such modalities as acupuncture, chiropractic adjustments, kinesiology, homeopathy, and herbal medicine being used on a daily basis. The timing for Dr. Heinerman's guide could not be more perfect.

John's delightful style and message is quite different from many of the existing books on holistic care for animals. As a medical anthropologist, he is quite a character and and his conversational way of being courageously outspoken about many controversial topics, is truly refreshing. While I personally may not agree with John on such topics as spaying and neutering or the efficacy of homeopathic therapies, I continue to salute John for tackling these issues head on and for being forever true to his own opinions, no matter how controversial they may be perceived.

In his book, John effectively addresses many of the important issues animals and people face day to day. John further strikes a cord, with a great deal of clarity, as he focuses needed attention on such areas as the feeding of organic, pesticide-free foods and the appropriate use of medicinal herbs. I was personally touched by his dedication to the spiritual purpose for animals and how they intertwine in our human–animal companion bond relationship, serving and teaching unconditionally—like a rich dessert following a special meal.

Whatever your motivation was in purchasing and reading John's book, I believe you have a really good guide to natural remedies for animals which include many topics that you won't find in the traditional "how to" or A to Z guides to healing. I also believe that the benefits of the information found in the book will support animals, people and the environment, in which we mutually cohabit.

—Robert S. Goldstein, VMD

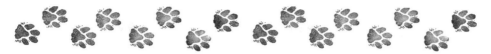

INTRODUCTION

Fifteen years ago I wrote a book entitled *Healing Animals with Herbs* (Provo, UT: BiWorld Publishers, Inc., 1983). It was a small but significant work of 117 pages. It covered all types of domesticated animals including some you wouldn't think of as being in the animal category or even qualifying as household pets: sheep, goats, cows, horses, poultry, bees, monkeys, hamsters, and rabbits. The briefest section was on cats and dogs and filled a mere three pages.

The book did a fairly brisk business selling about 27,000 copies in the two years it was in print. There were a few decent reviews and some very nice correspondence (mostly from farmers) thanking me for putting together a work that offered folks some natural alternatives to the chemical drugs being routinely used by veterinarians everywhere. Besides a couple of other books, mine was only one of about three or four devoted exclusively to animal care using herbs and other natural substances.

Fast-forward to 1998: An estimated 83 million Americans have at least one pet (usually a cat or dog) in their homes. The pet business today is currently a multibillion-dollar market. Explosive growth in organic pet foods and supplements is taking place within the huge health-food movement. And veterinarians by the number are realizing where the dollars are and incorporating many alternative methods into their regular medical practice. This is not to mention another business that caters to the exclusively well-heeled and rakes in millions of bucks in the process: pet jewelry, pet furs, pet pedicures, pet massages, pet saunas, and even pet vacations and pet hotels, if you can imagine!

There really seems to be no end to the extravagant lengths that owners will go to to pamper their prized animals, regardless of the cost. Certainly in the eyes of those who view canines and felines as ordinary mutts and mousers, such spending is obscene, if not sinful.

But appreciation is a fairly relative virtue and gets equated to such lofty levels only in the minds and hearts of genuine pet lovers. Like connoisseurs of fine wine or great cuisine, these folks measure true animal greatness in terms of the loyalty and devotion they receive to fill apparent emotional voids in their own lives. A survey in the May 1995 issue of *Veterinary Economics* reported that 60 percent of the cat owners in America paid as much attention to their cats as they did to their own kids. And 69 percent of the dog owners were just as concerned about their pets as their children.

When I started examining the book market to find what was out there on the subject, I was surprised to find only a mere handful of titles devoted exclusively to the theme of natural animal care. A couple were deemed worthy, a few mediocre, and the rest not worth the price of admission into their pages. Even then, I was mildly disappointed to discover in the several good books a lack of topics I felt were appropriate to an animal-care book. I mean, when was the last time *you* saw animal abandonment, anxiety, litterbox clumping, loneliness, or pain in a cat or dog book of any merit?

Another factor that gradually prodded me toward writing a volume such as this were the ever increasing demands from loyal fans to do something for their pets as I had done for them through the years with a multitude of other books. At book signings and public-speaking appearances, in letters, and through telephone calls from numerous people seeking additional health wisdom for this or that malady, I would invariably be asked questions pertaining to their favorite cat or dog. In time I came to be not only an expert in herbal folk medicine, nutrition, and food therapy, but also an unlicensed "vet at large." Having used natural substances for many years on our own farm animals and pets, as well as those of friends, neighbors, and staff, I was already pretty familiar with what items worked the best in a particular health stress or situation.

As inevitable forces of persuasion from all sides gently pushed me in the direction of writing a book such as this, I decided to "bone up" on those few areas I felt needed some further knowledge-fortifying. So I commenced getting some good (and expensive) veterinary works and reading them for any additional data I felt might be useful and might serve my readers well when undertaking this project. Besides this, I spoke with a number of veterinarians all across the country, some by phone, some through the mail, and some in person. I got a good cross-section of healing views that enabled me to expand my own treatment skills even more.

After all of this work and effort I felt it was time to undertake the task at hand. I included here without hesitation some of the product manufacturers I had used in previous books and knew to be reliable. But I still hadn't found any companies specifically serving the pet market that I could honestly recommend to my readers and still feel good about. After spending hours and hours walking what seemed to be miles of carpeted floor at several huge health-food industry convention shows and gathering armloads of printed information and free samples, I managed to compile a list of 15 such firms. But they say that the closer you examine something, the quicker it loses its appeal. I learned a hard lesson from all of my canvassing: You *cannot* believe what you read, are told, or see *most* of the time.

It became very discouraging to learn that so-called *natural* products were, in many instances, quite *un*natural. Talk about disillusionment! I was pretty disgusted at the end of my long investigative journey. I remember one night asking my aged father rather wearily, "Dad, why do *so* many deceive others?" And his pat reply was, "John, remember that's the type of world we're living in at present; did you expect anything different?" I then realized why he was exceedingly wise in his mid-eighties, while I was still in the pursuit of it in my early fifties.

Finally, almost providentially, I might add, I found a couple of companies whose pet products met my own self-imposed standards of excellence and reliability. After that, I slept better and wrote more gladfully. They weren't big and glitzy and lacked the deep corporate pockets of other animal needs' businesses. But their proprietors are principled people and what they make qualifies for the three E's: economical, effective, and ethical.

It would certainly come across to some as almost egotistical were I to declare on this page that my book is the definitive work on natural pet care. I don't believe (from everything else I've seen on the subject) that any book really qualifies for that kind of blue-ribbon assessment. But what I can say—and what probably more correctly reflects the mission of this book—is that it *truly* represents a *distillation* of healing wisdom from *numerous* sources. Think of my humble work as an "information center" of sorts, where pet owners can come to find general and specific data on many problems that afflict their cats and dogs. And in cases where additional data may be required, readers can refer themselves to Appendices II and III, wherein are given almost 30 different resource materials in the ways of books, magazines, and newsletters that they may reliably consult for whatever else is needed.

But my "clearinghouse" for data goes well beyond the written word or recorded fact. It goes to the heart and soul of why we keep animals around us in the first place. I wrote this book *because* I love animals, plain and simple! And any former or present pet owner who has formed an attachment of some sort with his or her favorite cat or dog will know exactly what I mean. There is a bond between pet and person that transcends even human levels. In some ways (and I hope I'm not misunderstood when I say this), this connection almost belongs in the metaphysical dimension.

The patience, loyalty, and devotion that small (and larger) animals give their masters is nothing short of incredible. And their companionships often mold and remake us in ways we do not know. While it is true that they garner our deepest affections and esteem, these wonderful creatures continually impart these priceless virtues of which we speak in measured doses over their lifetimes. As a result we (it's hoped) become better human beings because of them.

One is almost tempted to find a religious practice of some kind at work here. But lest I be accused of blasphemy in the extreme, I shall resist such further speculative contemplations. Still, I think, you will have to agree with me that the finest sermons ever given on patience, loyalty, and devotion weren't preached over the pulpit in man-made temples of worship. Instead, we are continually being inspired with our animals' importance in human life, every time our cats rub up against our legs and meow ever so sweetly and our dogs gratefully lick our hands and look at us through faithful eyes.

This, I sincerely believe, is how the Creator can more effectively get across to us the messages embodied in these three eternal virtues. He uses our animal companions to teach us truths no reverend divine or minister of the cloth could ever declare with such eloquence and piety.

—John Heinerman, Ph.D.

So Human an Animal

I look at kitty
And what do I see
But a part of me—
Its frolic and fun
Are humor and pun
For the jokes I've spun.

Rover, over there
Gives me patient stare
And kindly look fair.
In turn I should be
Same virtuously
To others, gladly.

—John Heinerman 1/31/98

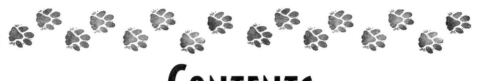

CONTENTS

Barking   39

Behavior Problems   42

Bladder Problems   55

Body Odors   57

Bruised Paws   61

Bumps & Bruises   63

Pain   231

Pancreatitis   245

Parasites   248

Paralysis   248

Paroviral Infection   254

Pet Therapy   255

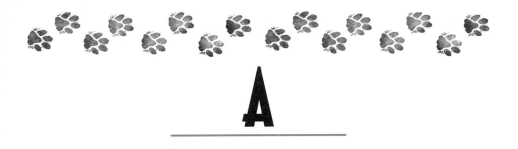

A

ABSCESS

Natural Treatment

Dr. Bob Goldstein and his wife, Susan, are two of America's most beloved and nationally known pet-care authorities. Bob holds a degree in veterinary medicine from the University of Pennsylvania, where they still give degrees in Latin—hence the VMD after his name. Susan is an expert on animal nutrition and the emotional well-being of cats and dogs. Her work has earned her coverage by *The New York Times,* the *Wall Street Journal,* NBC, and CBS. Together, they edit an internationally circulated health newsletter entitled *Love of Animals.*

The following information is from the September 1995 issue of that publication and is reproduced here with their kind permission. (See Appendix II for subscription information and Appendix III for contacting them in person.)

"If you find a fresh wound, gently rub the wound edges and pull out any hair or debris. Trim the surrounding hair away and clean the area with hydrogen peroxide. Then dress the wound with a dab of aloe vera gel. You can help your cat fight any infection by boosting the immune system. A cat with a strong, active immune system will resist infection and heal the area spontaneously. A less healthy animal may develop an abscess.

"Abscesses should be taken seriously, as they often lead to blood poisoning (septicemia), either locally or throughout the body. For a local infection, put your animal on this daily regimen:

Vitamin C—250 mg. three times daily

Bee Propolis—1/2 tablet twice daily

Garlic—1 capsule twice daily*

Echinacea—1 capsule daily

If you find an abscess, have your veterinarian drain the abscess and try this plan:

Vitamin C—500 mg. three times daily

Bee Propolis—1 tablet three times daily

Garlic—1 tablet three times daily*

Echinacea—1 capsule three times daily

Calendula—1/2 tsp. in cup of warm water; soak extremity or sore area."

*Consult the Product Appendix under Wakunage for the garlic brand that I recommend all the time.

(Also see Infection and Wounds for additional information.)

ALLERGIES

Allergy Inducements

An allergy is a physical manifestation of a weakened or damaged immune system reacting inappropriately to a harmless substance. It can also be a reaction to the body itself, as in the case of autoimmune disorders such as allergic dermatitis, asthma, irritable-bowel syndrome, and rheumatoid arthritis. But an allergy isn't a disease in and of itself.

Nature designed the immune system of humans and animals to protect the body from those substances that may irritate or damage it in some way. The immune response is directly tied in with the digestive system, which then rejects that item through vomiting or diarrhea. But if the substance being rejected is harmless, then it becomes an allergy.

Doctors of veterinary medicine (DVM) with some background in immunology and who practice along alternative lines of healing have indicated that allergies are a combination of several factors rather than just one thing. In a number of phone interviews I conducted with different DVMs around the country in mid-December 1997 on this topic, a variety of viewpoints emerged that I have consolidated into three major categories.

1. *Poor diet.* Many felt that the poor quality of food given to cats and dogs these days accounted for the majority of allergy cases they were seeing on a regular basis. This broke down into (a) excessive amounts of cooked (canned) food, (b) food containing chemical preservatives and artificial colorings, (c) and pet foods containing moldy grain or rancid meats.

The majority of interviewees concurred that *more raw food* was essential to the good health of cats and dogs. Raw food was more nutritious and could be better digested. Raw food contributed to the increase of enzymatic activities within the gut and bowels of such animals, making them look and feel healthier. Raw food strengthened the immune systems of such animals, enabling them to ward off infectious diseases more easily.

Also, raw-food diets prompted animals to eat *less.* Of the seventeen or so veterinarians who were kind enough to share some of their time with me by phone, eleven of them brought out this point, which I thought was highly interesting. Opinions differed, of course, as to how this might work. One California doctor believes that the high amount of mineral salts in a raw-food diet satisfies an animal's hunger better than does cooked (canned) food—in which case the animal doesn't have to eat as much. Another veterinarian ascribed the high fiber content present in raw foods to controlling the weight of household pets. He felt that with a lot of bulk roughage present in the animal's gut, the desire to eat more often and in greater quantities would be naturally curbed. A third animal-care practitioner stated flat-out that "since raw foods have life and vitality, the animal has more energy to run off the fat and carbohydrates so they don't accumulate on his body" with the passing of time.

2. *Vaccinations.* This was a prickly area of discussion for some DVMs, who still insisted (in spite of their holistic approaches) that *some* vaccinations were necessary. They pointed out that certain laws in their particular states mandated that pet owners get their animals immunized. One veterinarian thus queried responded without any hesitation, "You wouldn't want the readers of your book breaking the law by not having their pets immunized, now, would you?" I found only two veterinarians willing to express their opinions on this highly charged issue, provided I didn't use their names or the places they practiced in. The first doctor outright labeled *all* vaccines as "poisonous to an animal's immune system." The other veterinarian gave a more controversial opinion: "If pet owners *really* knew what vaccines did to the health of their pets and loved them, they wouldn't get them vaccinated . . . period!"

A larger number, though, were willing to concede that *multiple* vaccines (the giving of frequent or repeated vaccines) could compromise the immune systems of many animals. The collective consensus was that immune responses might become confused in being able to distinguish between harmful and benign substances if multiple vaccines were used. But they still believed that vaccinations were necessary if held within reason. Personally, I have *never* had any of my large or small domesticated animals vaccinated. My parents never had their children vaccinated, so why should I immunize my pets?

3. *Inbreeding.* Dr. Alfred Plechner, a California veterinarian, co-authored with freelance writer Martin Zucker (and self-published) a fascinating little book entitled *Pet Allergies: Remedies for an Epidemic* (Inglewood, CA: Very Healthy Enterprises, 1986) over a decade ago. This is what he says about the matter: "The recent history of cosmetic breeding practices among cat and dog breeders is replete with bad news—animals and gross deformities, lost instincts, altered and bizarre behavior and specific health problems."

As an anthropologist, I've examined inbreeding from human and plant perspectives. What I've found along the way may well be applicable when it comes to pets. The Amish people have inbred for many generations. As a consequence of their very small gene pool, a number of genetic birth defects and inherent medical weaknesses become evident with each new generation. And the selective growing of new hybrid plants for commercial purposes by giant agribusiness corporations results in crop species unable to survive in the wild. What all of this amounts to really is weakened stock.

It has been casually reported through numerous anecdotal stories that the "mongrel mix" or "Heinz 57" varieties of cats and dogs usually stand a much better chance of living long without incurring common health problems than do their cousins originating from purebred lines. While it is true that the alley cat or junkyard dog may never garner any blue-ribbon awards at pet shows, they each will thrive a lot better than those pampered pets with papered pedigrees a mile long.

These, then, are the three categories deemed most responsible for inducing the greater majority of allergies typically seen in household pets today.

Allergic Responses

A retired veterinarian told me some time ago that when he entered his profession as a young man in the early 1940s, "I hardly ever saw an allergic condition in any of the animals I treated." But with the advent of chemical pesticides and additives in modern agriculture and food manufacturing, "there has been a steady incline in allergies and immune-system problems." In fact, he said, "these became the most frequent conditions I treated in the last seven years prior to my retirement.

"Dogs express their allergic reactions much differently than cats do," he noted. A general itchiness of the skin and periodic rash or sores are common, "particularly in and around their tail areas." But they aren't just confined to this region and can show up anywhere else for that matter. Dogs with allergies typically suffer from inflammation of the ears, toes, and genitals. There is usually frequent gastrointestinal disturbance marked by gurgling sounds in the stomach, discharged gas, and runny stool.

Cats also experience skin eruptions when they're allergic to something that show up in the form of an animal dermatitis. They are, by far, more subject to bladder inflammation and digestive upset than dogs are. Many times cats won't even display any external evidence on their skin indicating allergic responses. But the stinging sensations they feel internally will cause erratic behavior in them: They will be quite fidgety, nervously licking themselves, and periodically biting themselves. Their strange actions would seem to suggest the presence of fleas, but they are, in fact, really *undetected allergies.*

Control Tips

There are some things that a pet owner can do to bring comfort to a small animal suffering from the symptoms of an allergy. Those that are nondietary are mentioned here; those that involve specific food changes are listed separately.

I've discovered through the years that nothing seems to benefit the skin manifestations of an animal's allergy more than by giving it a gentle bath. Tap water should *not* be used for this purpose because of the chlorine and fluoride it may contain. Instead, an adequate amount of distilled, purified, or spring water should be heated until lukewarm. Gauge the amount needed by the size of the animal: Animals under ten inches in height need no more than a gallon at most, while those taller than this may require up to several gallons.

Use a very mild soap when washing the animal. You *don't* want something containing a lot of chemicals that would only further irritate the existing allergic condition. The best place to look in a large department store, supermarket, or pharmacy is in the section that sells baby items. There you can find a baby shampoo that should work effectively. Afterwards, rinse the animal's coat or skin several times with an equal mixture of *cool* water (not tap) and tincture of witch hazel. You can also substitute cool, strained peppermint tea in place of the witch hazel, if you like.

In those areas of the skin where the animal has scratched or bitten itself frequently, you should apply cold herbal compresses. Use an old piece of sheet or washrag for this that has been laundered without any soap and dried. Soak the material in some cool peppermint tea, wring out the excess liquid, fold over, and apply to the affected area. Preferably, the animal should be lying down and you should hold the compress in place for several minutes while speaking to your pet. Not only will the herbal compress promote healing of the skin, but you will also be able to better bond with the animal as well. The affected area can also be sprayed with tincture of witch hazel following several compress treatments.

In a few more severe cases, you may need to apply a paste to those areas of the skin that have been previously bitten or scratched in order to promote healing. Mix one tablespoon of baking soda with one-half teaspoon each of powdered Echinacea and goldenseal. Then add just enough distilled or filtered water to make a paste that can be put on with a tongue depressor or some other flat object.

An animal's hind quarters may be sprayed with a solution of hyssop and peppermint or with witch hazel combined with either of those herbs. Just make a simple tea by steeping one teaspoon of hyssop *or* peppermint leaves in one-half pint boiling water. When cool, strain the liquid and combine it with one-half cup of tincture of witch hazel that can be purchased from any supermarket or pharmacy. Put this in an empty spray bottle and squirt some around the animal's anus to relieve itching and inflammation. One teaspoon of each herb in one pint of boiling water, simmered for 15 minutes, strained, and cooled before bottling is equally effective. Other areas of the body that show allergic symptoms may also be sprayed with this herbal solution.

Aloe-vera gel works surprising well for allergic skin responses that have been chewed on, frequently licked, or continually scratched. However, before applying aloe to the affected area, I suggest adding two drops of wormwood or valerian tea. You need only a little amount of either herb, no more than one-half teaspoons steeped in one-half cup boiling water for ten minutes, covered, to get the desired results. Both herbs have a nasty taste to them and when a few drops are added to the aloe gel before application, it's guaranteed to stay on the skin. If the animal attempts to lick it off, it is in for a flavorful surprise!

Helpful Tea for an Allergic Cat

A tea I developed for one pet owner about 15 years ago helped her deal with a finicky Persian cat that was suffering from irritated eyes and inflamed ears due to allergic reactions. I had her mix one teaspoon each of eyebright herb, red-raspberry leaves, and stinging nettle herb and steep in one-and-a-half pints boiling distilled water for 15 minutes.

The cool tea was then strained and put into a spray bottle. It was a bit tricky spraying some of this solution into her cat's face and making sure she got the eyes, nose, and ears. She required some assistance from her husband in holding the animal down while this was done. After a while, she found it easier to bathe these parts with this solution using a cotton swab; the animal offered less resistance this way.

A Tucson, Arizona, company offers several products to assist animals with allergic reactions. Consult the Product Appendix under Holistic Animal Care for more information.

Good Diet Is the Key to Successful Allergy Management

At the end of 1997 I celebrated my fifty-first birthday (December 3). For most of my life, I have regularly consumed cooked oatmeal every morning for breakfast. About the only times I've missed this routine is when I've had to travel to exotic places (South Sea islands) or remote corners of the world (Mongolia) for research or speaking purposes. Then I've had to settle for whatever else was available, ranging from cooked poi with coconut milk to boiled rice and yak butter.

It took me many years, though, before I finally made a connection between oatmeal consumption and a virtual absence of those symptoms commonly connected with hay fever or asthma. I've never used sugar, honey, or fruit juice to sweeten my oatmeal, preferring to eat it plain with just a little milk. But the apparent protection that this particular cereal grain afforded me seems to carry over to household animals as well.

Below are two simple diets, one for a cat and the other for a dog, that will help an animal recover from an allergy. Only distilled, filtered, or spring water should be used in their preparations. The animal should be kept on it for a minimum of six weeks. After this, the pet owner should be judicious in selecting the right kind of food that will continue to promote good health in the animal. (Check the Product Appendix under Holistic Animal Care for a good brand of wholesome pet food that can be trusted.)

The meat to be used in the preparation of either recipe should be certified organic. In some parts of the country, Coleman Natural Products are available at larger health-food stores with meat departments. With this label, you are always guaranteed to get meat that is completely free of chemical additives. *This is important to remember* when shopping for beef or mutton, since a major part of an animal's existing allergies may be attributed to the accumulated chemical residues within its system from the commercial food it previously ate.

The particular supplement I recommend should be added only at the time of feeding. It should *never* be mixed in during the actual meal preparation. For an average cat, three tablets should be crushed into powder with a heavy object and added to the food just before serving. For a small- to medium-sized dog, six tablets should be crushed and added prior to the food that will be eaten. Most of the nutrients in this supplement formula come from the Great Salt Lake and are designed to add luster, beauty, and strength to the hair, skin, and nails of pets and pet owners alike. (Look for the product name of With-In under Trace Minerals Research in the Product Appendix.)

ANTI-ALLERGY DIET (CATS)

8 cups nonchlorinated/nonfluoridated water

4 cups rolled oats

4 cups organic beef or mutton

1½ teaspoons bonemeal

2 tablespoons canola oil

With-In mineral-vitamin supplement

Boil the water in a stainless-steel or glass pan. Add the oats and cook 12 minutes, stirring occasionally. The consistency should be thick and soft or somewhat mushy.

Remove excess fat from the meat. Using a large knife with a sharp blade, cut the meat into very tiny pieces or run it through a grinder. (The electric kind is obviously the quickest and easiest. But the kind you can clamp to the edge of a table or counter is just as good, though more manual labor is involved.)

Mix the meat pieces in with the cooked mush. Cool. This should feed a hungry adult cat for about a week. Some of it can be put into a plastic storage bowl with a lid and frozen to prevent spoilage, if necessary. With each feeding, warm up a little, then stir in the mineral-vitamin powder from three crushed tablets before serving.

ANTI-ALLERGY DIET (DOGS)

4½ quarts water (not from the tap)
10 cups rolled oats
4¼ cups organic *beef or mutton*
3 teaspoons bonemeal
½ cup canola oil
Within-In mineral-vitamin supplement

Boil the water in a pot or pan other than aluminum. Add the oats and cook 12 minutes, stirring periodically until a mushy consistency is reached. Trim the meat of excess fat, then finely mince or grind. Add it to the mush and allow contents to cool. This should be enough to feed a small- to medium-sized dog for five days. Refrigerate or freeze what you don't use.

To every feeding, add the powder from six crushed tablets of the mineral-vitamin formula.

Also see under Itching and Skin Problems for additional information.

What to Do When You Become Allergic to Your Animal

It is a common fact that people who are allergic to small animals with lots of fur or hair will still keep them on their premises in spite of the health consequences. I know this to be true, because for almost five years I suffered (as did my staff) when our mixed Persian-Siamese cat named Jake had free run of Anthropological Research Center. When we relocated and Jake went to the family farm in southern Utah, I quickly discovered how much easier it was for me to breathe again. And people who knew me from before now remarked, "Looks like you finally got over your long head cold" or "Well, your years-long sinus problem seems to have cleared up at last."

The obvious health risks to harboring a pet (especially a cat) to which you may be allergic includes asthma, bronchitis, emphysema, hay fever, and similar respiratory stresses. But according to a fairly recent study, at least one third of Americans who are allergic to pets (mostly felines) live with a least one of them in their dwellings. That figures out to be about two million noses, which is no small problem to be sneezing at.

Allergies to pets pose awful consequences: sneezing, runny eyes, perpetual stuffed noses, and dangerous asthma attacks. The culprit in cats, of course, are glands within the skin that secrete minute allergy-triggering proteins called "allergens." These linger most abundantly in the cat's neck fur, but also float easily into the air. Allergens are likewise present in the animal's saliva and urine. Once a cat has licked itself, the saliva on the fur dries and microscopic bits of this chip off and soon become airborne. It is important to note that the cat's hair doesn't in itself provoke an allergenic reaction. All in all, having a cat around means having plenty of cat allergen as well.

With dogs, it's nowhere near as bad, since they don't lick themselves as much as cats do. But some of the more hairy breeds can in time trigger allergic responses of their own if they're allowed to go for very long periods without suitable bathing.

A psychologist at the University of British Columbia in Western Canada evaluated 341 pet owners who were allergic to their cats or dogs and had been counseled by their respective physicians to give up their animals. Only one out of five did. Furthermore, when 122 lost their pets, 70 percent of them went out and promptly got replacements. The implication seems clear enough: The pet is more important in terms of lifestyle and needs than is the alleviation of medical symptoms.

While washing the pet frequently seems to be a logical solution, in other ways it isn't. Most cats detest water, and dogs aren't too crazy about it either. A weekly wash followed by immersion in comfortably warm (100-degree) water did reduce allergens by 84 percent in one study, but only for a week. So unless you're prepared to bathe Kitty or Rover twice weekly, pet washing may not be the full answer to your allergy problems.

So let's look at priorities here. Doctors who specialize solely in allergies and pulmonary disorders strongly emphasize that if you have severe asthma, your pet *must* go or else you're apt to have a serious reaction a lot sooner than you may be prepared for. Beyond that, however, all other pet owners may retain their animals, but should follow these few simple suggestions to minimize the health side effects:

- Keep one area of your residence allergen-free (say, the bed-room). This means "off limits" to pets—*no* exceptions.

- Use a high-efficiency particulate air-HEPA cleaner in this room.

- Remember to close the door to your designated pet-free room upon entering and leaving.

- Use impermeable covers (encasements) for the mattress and pillow because they are tremendous reservoirs for allergens to accumulate.

- Remove any carpeting from your pet-free room. Try to have only wooden floors or tile instead. You'd be surprised at just how much difference this makes: The reduction of airborne allergens could be as great as 90 percent.

- Use a type of vacuum cleaner that has multiple filters for con-trolling airborne allergens. (See Product Appendix under Vita-Mix for information on their Vita-Vac cleaning machine.)

- If outside air is tolerable and the room has a window, keep it cracked a bit to let in fresh air periodically. Do not do this, however, if outside air is extremely polluted.

- Curtail the intake of sugar-rich foods and your allergenic responses will be cut in half.

ANAL INFLAMMATION

What to Do for a Sore Anus

A household pet will frequently get an inflamed anus due to many watery or loose stools. This causes the surrounding tissue to become irritated and occasionally infected with bacteria. A good hygienic practice during the diarrhea phase of a sickness is to moisten a clean cotton cloth slightly with a little distilled water and then to sponge the anus gently until it is free of debris.

Pat it dry with another clean cloth or some cotton balls. After this, take two or three cotton swabs, and holding them together in one hand, dip into a small amount of extra-virgin olive oil that has been poured into a small bowl made of paper or foil (for discarding later on). Slightly press out some of the excess oil before applying it to that area of the body. Repeat this procedure morning, noon, and night.

In the event a slight infection has occurred along with the inflammation, soak a couple of cotton swabs in a little *alcohol-free* liquid goldenseal-root extract and then dab around the anus. Do this several times a day for a few days until it looks as if the infection has gone away.

You can also apply one of several herbal creams that have great healing potential for such a condition. I recommend arnica or calendula creams for this purpose. (See Product Appendix under Nature's Answer for information on obtaining any of the items previously mentioned.)

ANEMIA

Associated with Numerous Diseases

Anemia is a common clinical sign associated with numerous diseases in animals and humans alike. The condition may be due to one or several of the following conditions:

- A reduction below normal in the number of red blood cells per cubic millimeter
- A drop in the quantity of oxygen-carrying pigment (hemoglobin) within such blood cells
- A decrease in the volume of packed red cells per 100 milliliters of blood, which occurs when equilibrium between blood loss (through bleeding or cell destruction) and blood production is disturbed in any way

Types and Signs

Veterinarians are acquainted with at least seven varieties of anemia:

1. Aplastic pancytopenia occurs in both dogs and cats.

2. Hemolytic anemia (Heinz body) is more common in cats than in dogs.

3. Immune mediated anemia affects dogs more than cats. Some breeds, in particular, are more susceptible to it: old English sheepdog, cocker spaniel, poodle, Irish setter, English springer spaniel, and border collie.

4. Iron-deficiency anemia is fairly evident in adult dogs, but seldom diagnosed in adult cats.

5. Megalobastic anemia can be a spontaneous event in dogs (toy poodles especially) and cats (those infected with feline leukemia).

6. Anemia due to chronic kidney disease affects most middle-aged to older dogs and cats, but is occasionally seen in younger animals, as well.

7. Metabolic anemia or spiculated red cells is fairly certain to occur in dogs with diseases of the liver and kidneys and infrequently in cats with fatty liver syndrome.

The most common signs of any form of anemia are lethargy, weakness, lack of appetite, breathing that is quick and shallow, weight loss, cold intolerance, apathy, depression, mood changes, excessive heartbeat, joint pain, occasional reddish-brown urine, and white (or pale) gums.

Animal anemias may be due to blood loss incurred from wounds, infections such as leukemia, or parasites such as fleas and worms. (For more specific information see under the individual entries for each: Feline Leukemia, Fleas, and Worms.)

Nutritional Support

Certain foods and supplements are critical to the body's reversing this problem by enhancing the production of healthy red blood cells. Organic beef, sheep, or chicken livers top the list because of their rich amino acids, B-complex (especially B-12), and iron contents. This should always be given *raw*—never cooked. Between the years 1932 and 1942, Dr. Francis M. Pottenger conducted extensive and long-range testing on numerous cats. Those felines who were fed only cooked meat in spite of an otherwise properly balanced diet showed classic symptoms of anemia and damaged immune systems. However, Dr. Pottenger was able to reverse these and other problems simply by returning the cats to a raw-food diet.

Under the entry for Anorexia, I discuss a Multipurpose Pet Puree that is beneficial for dogs and cats. The centerpiece of nourishment is raw organic liver along with other ingredients. Details are provided on how to make it using a Vita-Mix 5000 machine. (See Appendix I for information about this product.) Desiccated liver tablets and powdered liver can also be used if necessary. These supplements may be obtained at most health-food stores, pet-supply centers, or some veterinarians.

Brewer's yeast is a useful item and duplicates some of the same nutritional benefits that liver does. But due to its smell or taste, it might be better to mix a little in with the animal's food: one-half tablespoon for small and one-and-a-half tablespoons for large-sized animals.

Certain grains and vegetables have respectable amounts of iron and other minerals that are important to the blood-rebuilding process. These include pumpkin, Swiss chard, peas, collard greens, beet root and beet greens, lima beans, and mustard greens. Figs, raisins, and blackstrap molasses are good sources of this mineral, too, as are oatmeal and tofu. Some of these items should be lightly cooked and pureed before serving: pumpkin, oatmeal, beets, and lima beans. Others may be juiced in a blender: Swiss chard, collard greens, beet greens, and mustard greens. Commercially prepared tofu can be fed to an animal, but it is best to flavor it with a little blackstrap molasses. I would puree figs and raisins before serving them to an animal, since there is the risk of choking if they are swallowed without being chewed. A nice beet-juice powder and mixed greens are available, which can be reconstituted with water (see Product Appendix under Pines).

Sea vegetation is very good for correcting anemia as it contains myriad trace elements, including iodine, a mineral seldom found in land-grown plants. Kelp, dulse, kombu, nori, arame, wakame, and others make tasty dishes for discriminating pets' tastes. Some of them, such as kelp, are available as powders or granules and can easily be mixed with an animal's regular food. Or they can be made into flavorful soups, which animals and their owners should both enjoy a lot.

Dulse Soup

¼ cup dried dulse

1 cup parsnips or 1 cup carrots, diced

1 quart water

Chop the dried dulse coarsely. Boil the carrots or parsnips in the water until tender. Add the chopped dulse. Cook on medium heat for 12 minutes. Remove and permit to cool before serving your pet half the amount; refrigerate the rest for another meal later on.

Wakame and Split Pea Soup

1 cup dried split peas

1 ½ cups water

¼ cup dried wakame, crumbled

1 carrot, thinly sliced in rounds

2 tablespoons sesame-seed paste

pinch of sea salt

Simmer the split peas in water until tender, about 1 hour. Add the crumbled wakame and carrot. Cover and simmer to a creamy consistency, about 35 minutes longer. Set aside and stir in sesame-seed paste. Add salt to taste. Serve half this amount when cooled to lukewarm; refrigerate the rest for another meal.

Vitamin C, folic acid, and vitamin B-12 are necessary nutrients for treating animal anemia. They may be given in supplement form, preferably tablets, provided these are crushed to powder and mixed in with an animal's regular food. Small animals could use 500 mg. of vitamin C, 150 micrograms of folic acid, and 10 micrograms of vitamin B-12. For larger-sized pets, these amounts can be doubled.

Liver and brewer's yeast are good sources of vitamin B-12, while certain dark leafy vegetables such as broccoli, spinach, and romaine have adequate amounts of folic acid in them. It is best to lightly steam them, however, prior to serving, since it is difficult for animals to consume them in a raw state. A number of fresh fruits and vegetables have varying amounts of vitamin C in them. Animals may prefer some over others. With a little practice, an owner can determine which ones his or her pet likes or doesn't like.

ANIMAL ABANDONMENT

An Alarming Trend

I seldom watch TV talk shows, esteeming most of them as so much empty-headed nonsense or sensationalism broadcast for ratings appeal. However, on the day following Christmas, Friday, December 26, 1997, I happened to have my set turned on as I ate breakfast and read the morning newspaper.

The program then in progress was the talk show *Leeza,* out of Hollywood, hosted by Leeza Gibbons. Much of the time, she is notorious for having guests whose life stories are generally filled with perversion, violence, and abuse. But on this day, the sleaze was absent and in its place were heart-warming stories of pet adoptions from the local animal shelter in Los Angeles.

A statistic attributed to Doris Day was given during the show: Over 12 million dogs and cats are regularly put to sleep throughout animal pounds across America. (In recent years this aging screen star has become an outspoken critic of animal abandonment and has been actively involved in the placement of many of these animals in good homes.)

Several noted authorities from well-known animal shelters gave their views as to why this seems to be a growing problem throughout the country. The number-one reason many people gave for turning their pets into a shelter to be disposed of was moving. They didn't want to take their animals with them or else simply didn't have room in their new locations for them. The second most common reason cited was growth size: Many pet owners were unprepared for just how large their dogs eventually became after reaching full maturity. As one lady put it to a worker after dumping off four Dalmatians at a local pound: "They looked so much smaller *in the movie!*" She was obviously referring to the 1996 live action Disney holiday hit, *101 Dalmatians,* starring Glenn Close.

A third factor was economics: "Many pet lovers on budgets are finding out that their small animals are too expensive to feed," one official noted. "They're barely able to feed themselves or their families and then have to shell out bucks for dog or cat food. They often end up having to make tough choices that seem cruel by some people's standards."

Another thing that ranks up there for reasons of abandonment is, believe it or not, lack of interest in taking care of the animal after a while. This is especially true in young families with small children and is more common around Christmas and Easter than at any other time of the year. Well-meaning parents go out and buy their little tykes a cute kitten or puppy from a local pet store. The kids are enamored with their "live presents," because such small pets are cuddly and playful. What parents fail to understand, however, is that such animals require *daily* maintenance: feeding, watering, and cleaning up, not to mention a certain amount of time socially interacting with them.

Children's attention spans are incredibly short, and they grow bored of something in a hurry. The novelty of "newness" doesn't take long to wear off, and soon such pets become "yesterday's has-beens." Busy parents trying to juggle myriad activities then take on the additional responsibilities of caring for their youngsters' pets. After a brief stint of this, they fall prey to the easy temptation of abandonment and decide it's not worth the extra hassle to keep that loving cat or dog any longer.

One final category that can collectively be described only as "miscellaneous" involves one-of-a-kind or seldom heard reasons why some folks surrender their pets to the pound. One affluent couple who dropped their pair of eight-year-old, tan-colored cocker spaniels off at the L.A. Animal Shelter exclaimed that they had just redecorated their house in a new black-and-white motif, and that their dogs simply *"didn't match the décor"* anymore!

A Sensitive Topic Too Often Ignored

On the same program of *Leeza* was a renowned psychologist who specializes in human–small-animal relationships. It was her opinion that there would be considerably less abandonment if prospective owners first took a little "time out" and gave some serious thought as to what they were really getting themselves into. The pros and cons to animal ownership must be carefully weighed and *"truly legitimate"* reasons must be established for the acquisition of a pet.

Unless this is methodically done, people end up doing such animals only a "total disservice." "With acquisition there *must* be a real commitment of love *and* dedication toward the care of that pet," this psychologist emphasized. "Otherwise, the animal faces eventual abandonment, but sometimes in ways other than turning over to a pound." She cited a case of a wealthy family who took a lot of vacations and left the care of their several small household pets to the maid, chauffeur, and groundskeeper. After a while, during one of their brief trips home, they wondered why their favorite cats and dog no longer came running to them as before when called, but now seemed more to enjoy being around their hired help.

And a well-known Hollywood animal groomer, who was on the show to do complete "makeovers" for several pound mutts of mixed breeds, mentioned that most of the current books on natural care for household animals failed to include sections on animal abandonment. "It is a very touchy subject for many people," he admitted. "I have to be careful what I say to a good customer who is thinking of dumping his or her pet at the local shelter." A number of pet owners apparently get a guilt complex when contemplating such a thing. This is good for them to experience, for then they won't be so apt to abandon animals as easily.

Match the Pet with Owner's Personality

Of all the helpful suggestions given by a variety of guests on this edition of *Leeza,* none seemed so useful or sensible as the one put forward by the psychologist. "The best way to avoid this type of situation from ever occurring," she stated, "is for the pet of choice to be matched with the personality of the prospective buyer. Grumpy old men may get along better with bulldogs than French poodles." The audience laughed as she continued: "Little old ladies may prefer docile tabby cats instead of high-strung Chihuahuas."

Her point was well taken. A person needs to survey himself or herself and find out, first of all, "*Why* do I want a pet?" After that comes an honest introspection of personal moods, likes and dislikes, and unique or unusual personality quirks. Then the individual should consult with an animal expert of some kind—someone who is intimately familiar with the traits and habits of the animal being considered for purchase or adoption. This doesn't necessarily need to be an animal psychologist. It can be a professional breeder, a veterinarian, a groomer, or even an animal-shelter worker. All of them are well qualified to offer expert opinions on the animals available.

Once mental input has been made of that information, a "sorting-out" process follows whereby the prospective owner should be able to reflect on what animal characteristics best match his or her own personality traits. If this process is performed correctly and meditatively and not in haste, the individual should be able to choose correctly the kind of cat or dog that will provide many years of loving companionship for both parties.

I recommend that the reader turn to the entry under loneliness and read the data there concerning the potential negative health impacts that loneliness can have upon a household pet. Between the two sections, a person should receive enough guidance in order to select wisely and safely the kind of animal that will bring happiness and joy for a long time to come.

A Nation Gone (Literally) to the Dogs

If the stray pooches in your city are of a bothersome nature or social concern to you, you might want to consider yourself fortunate that you don't live in the capital of the former Communist-bloc country Romania. If Rome is famous for its pope and stray cats and New

York City for its outspoken lawyer-mayor and rats, then Bucharest is renowned for its gross mismanagement and dogs—lots of them, as a matter of fact. An estimated one-quarter *million* mangy mutts roam the city, cowering in doorways, dashing in front of cars, foraging for food, and biting whoever or whatever gets in their way.

The problem is so bad that when First Lady Hillary Rodham Clinton visited there in 1996, a large pack of mongrels estimated to be near 150 in number chased away the brave security guards who were scoping an area around a hospital just before her arrival. Fortunately for her, the guards returned with reinforcements and shot dead some 37 dogs before the rest dispersed helter-skelter.

The dogs saunter along the sidewalks with a confident air, sniffing around for scraps and rooting through garbage cans at night. The bites they inflict tend to be more painful than dangerous. Bucharest hasn't had a recorded case of rabies since 1969. But citizens still get the shots as a precaution.

After the shooting incident with the pack that threatened the First Lady's arrival, local authorities proposed a wholesale killing of other strays. But when word of this idea leaked to the foreign press, a small international storm of protest occurred. Even retired French actress Brigitte Bardot got into the act and contacted Bucharest's mayor to plead for canine clemency. Opposition parties exploited the issue, accusing the mayor of having an icy heart; residents told local and foreign reporters that killing the dogs would violate Christian values.

So the only thing left to do was for the metropolitan dog catchers (there are eight of them) to round up what strays they could, impound them for medical checkups and sterilization, then turn them loose again. After this surgical procedure, they tend not to be so aggressive. The city originally had three trucks in service, but a third was put out of commission in December 1997 when a pack of dogs chewed up the engine wiring from *beneath* the truck.

[I am grateful to Nicolae Radek of Bucharest for sending me clippings of articles on this subject from two major newspapers, *Adevârul (The Truth)* and *Romania Liebera (Free Romania)* as well as the English translations for them.]

ANIMAL AGGRESSION

The Territorial Factor

Cats and dogs, like many of their owners, can be territorial to some degree. This means that they identify with a certain amount of space, be it inside a house or an apartment or outside in a yard. Anyone whom they don't recognize or like intruding into that space will receive an unmistakable hiss or growl, suggesting the individual back off and go elsewhere.

A few species of animals, like some people, will be more territorial in nature than others. Persian cats and pit bulls are apt to defend their spaces far more aggressively than, say, a feline of mixed breed or a border collie might do. Such animals require areas that are securely fenced in or else must be placed on strong leashes (more so for the dogs than cats).

Trained That Way

Sometimes it becomes necessary for dogs to be trained to respond aggressively to certain situations. Anyone who has ever watched episodes from the real-life TV drama hit *Cops,* on the Fox Network, will know just how quickly various police K-9 corps have gone into action to apprehend a suspect the police are after for a crime committed.

In other instances, guard dogs are frequently used by some businesses during night hours to reduce burglaries and other unwanted intrusions. Such dogs are very alert and usually in a state of medium tension at all times. When necessary, they can spring into rapid action to meet the challenges at hand.

Such behavior is expected by their handlers. Dogs such as these go through rigorous training to develop an aggression that's strictly controlled by those humans with whom they are assigned to work. This aggression is part of their professional performance and comes into play when warranted. Otherwise, the animals are taught to hold it in check.

Prevention Is the First Line of Defense

Never assume that a "nice" cat or dog will always remain that way. Animal moods, just like human ones, may vary on a daily or even an *hourly* basis. That cat whose fur you rubbed in the morning may rake your ankle or hand later in the day. And a lovable pat on Rover's head in the afternoon might result in a bite at night.

There are numerous causes for such animal aggression. One can be physiological. There is a developing theory within veterinary medicine that there is an animal equivalent of human hypoglycemia, which results in drastic mood swings when blood-sugar levels fall below normal. Also, another common disorder is chronic encephalitis, which is behind a great many canine misbehaviors. This inflammation of the nervous system can be attributed to an autoimmune disorder or negative reactions to vaccinations. Canine and feline distempers, which are caused by canine distemper virus and feline parovirus, also are known to induce strange behavior and unanticipated aggressions.

If any of these factors are suspected, the pet should be taken to the veterinarian as soon as possible. There, a thorough examination can be done and tests run if necessary in order to determine if the aggression is physiologically based. It is often easier for people to identify something such as hypoglycemia or viral-induced fever in themselves than in their pets. That's why a trip to the vet becomes necessary under such suspicious circumstances.

Being on the lookout for things that might induce sudden aggression in animals and seeing that they don't occur is another good approach. Animals react instantly when suddenly startled. In their surprised states they're obviously going to react with anger, and not always in a very nice way. Think back to the last time you were frightened by something and how your reacted. Animals are no different in this respect.

Teasing is a big cause of animal aggression. Children and teenagers who themselves may manifest antisocial traits are the biggest culprits in this area. Sometimes a dog will put up with having its ears pulled or tail tugged by very small children. But at other times, when the dog is not feeling well or wishes to eat its food in peace, it may turn around and nip some of the little tormentors.

Unfortunately in such situations, adults overreact and the dog is either severely punished, locked up, or even put to sleep.

Hugging a cat or dog too long is another way of provoking unpleasant reactions. A pet may want to be free, but is still being restrained. Its only natural recourse is to scratch and bite in order to wiggle free. It has that right to do so, although the human smothering it with affection may think differently.

Household pets get highly excitable when their owners become excitable. I remember a couple of years ago I got into a heated argument with one of my secretaries over a job-related matter. In the course of our screaming and shouting, my office cat Jake walked by us and started meowing loudly. I looked down momentarily and shouted in anger, "Oh, shut up!" He hissed back. In return I scooted him aside with my foot. B-A-D mistake!

Jake turned suddenly and raked my one foot with his claws before running under the desk and away from me. Immediately, my secretary and I stopped our arguing and tended to my wound. The gash went pretty deep into the leg muscles and we had to use hydrogen peroxide and iodine to cleanse and treat the wound before bandaging it. I then turned my attention back to my cat and attempted to call him out from behind a bookcase in fake tones of niceness. But he wasn't fooled at all and remained behind there for several hours until he felt sure I had calmed down and was more kindly disposed toward him again.

It took a number of weeks for my lacerations to heal. But with ample intakes of Kyolic garlic, vitamins A, C, and E, and goldenseal root every day, I managed to come out of it all right without incurring infection or even having to see a doctor about it. The moral to this little tale, of course, is obvious: Don't yell or wave your hands around cats or dogs. They'll react in ways you won't like—*guaranteed!*

Show No Fear and Be Watchful

An animal's body language usually indicates the mood it is in at any given time. If it's in a friendly mood, there will be very little direct eye contact. The mouth will be open, almost in the form of a grin sometimes. The ears lie flat, the tail is tucked down or swishing from side to side, and the body is crouched low. This is when he or she is the most playful and poses no immediate threat.

But, on the other hand, there are enough signs to be on the lookout for when the same animal is in a potentially bad mood. The ears may be flat or sometimes raised up and forward. The lips are drawn back into a snarl or a hiss, revealing bare teeth. The hair or fur is raised high on the shoulders and rump. As the level of anger intensifies, the cat or dog in question may become stiff-legged, raising one front paw, hissing or growling, warily looking you in the eyes, and ever so slowly waving a high, arched tail. In such a stance, it must be clearly understood that this animal *means business* and is to be left alone at all costs.

Not all species give advance notice of "bad-hair" (or fur) days, trying to read them may be futile. Siamese cats, pit bulls, and chows are particularly notorious this way, and extreme caution needs to be used in dealing with them.

In the event that a larger pet such as a big dog runs toward you in a hostile way, *do not* exhibit fear. Animals can "smell" or detect it at a great distance. That gives them an immediate advantage over you, making them act more boldly as the aggressors and making you behave more like a victim.

Remain calm. Turn sideways a little and speak in a soft, soothing voice. Keep your head slightly bent and your hands by your sides. The angry dog can then see that this conveys peaceable intentions. Under no circumstances should you ever face the canine head-on or stare it down. That will only prompt a quicker attack.

And never turn and run away unless you are absolutely certain that you can get to safety in plenty of time. The genetically inherited wolflike tendencies of larger dogs is to view running creatures as escaping prey. Their natural instincts will be to want to give chase or attempt to bring it down.

Whistling softly or speaking gently to the animal will keep its mind occupied with the thought of possible peace. At the same time, you may wish to walk sideways or backwards ever so slowly in order to get to safety. Even singing a favorite hymn has been known to "soothe the savage beast" in man and animal alike on occasion. I've used it a couple of times myself over the years when confronted by someone else's mean mongrel.

Improving Animal Emotions

An animal's mental and emotional well-being is just as important as that of its master. When a pet is well-adjusted, there is virtually no display of aggressive behavior. In addition to the more obvious methods of displaying physical affection, giving plenty of verbal encouragement and compliments, and spending as much time as possible with your pet, there are herbal solutions for improving an animal's disturbed emotions.

Cats and dogs that have a tendency to manifest fear will benefit greatly from flower essences. These help to gradually remove anxieties and other emotional imbalances by creating a chemical confidence within. Star of Bethlehem and arnica are wonderful in dealing with past traumas, including kitten or puppy abandonment and physical abuse. Rock rose is especially useful for dealing with cases of animal panic.

Individual herbal liquid extracts that are alcohol-free also have a great effect in dispelling animal aggression before it gets out of hand. I would recommend without hesitation linden flower, wood betony, hops, and catnip (for cats mostly), peppermint, chamomile, or valerian. Also a combination of several of these herbs helps to reduce tension. (Consult the Product Appendix under Nature's Answer for more about these herbs.)

The standard dosages for such liquid extracts to be administered internally are as follows:

- One-half teaspoon three times daily for cats and dogs weighing less than 20 pounds
- One teaspoon three times daily for dogs weighing between 20 and 40 pounds
- One tablespoon three times daily for dogs weighing more than 40 pounds

They can be given orally by prying the animal's mouth open with one *gloved* hand and pouring the herbal liquids in with the other. Or else try to add it to some of the pet's water supply. Filling an eyedropper with the prescribed amount and squirting it into the animal's mouth is usually a bit easier than trying to pour it down with a spoon.

Many times stress can be massaged out of an animal before it turns into hostile aggression. Begin with a soft pat on the head and gentle rubbing around the eyes and on the face. Then stroke the back of the neck and underneath it. Now rub both hands along the top of the animal's spine toward the rump. Repeat this simple procedure, but this time slide the hands over each side. On the next trip around glide one hand or both under the belly toward the back legs. After this, stroke each leg in turn and then the tail as well. Go back to rubbing the ears, which all animals seem to enjoy a lot. You'll be amazed at just how much this helps. In addition, it gives you the added benefit of interacting with your pet in a positive and meaningful way. With treatment such as this, your animal should have no cause for serious aggression, beyond little moments of frustration common to every cat and dog in existence.

ANOREXIA

Common to Many Life Forms

The lack or loss of appetite for food is common to most life forms. From the titmouse (a bird) to a monstrous whale, many creatures that fly, swim, or walk will abstain from food for certain periods of time if they are not feeling well. This is an almost automatic response built into their systems by nature. Those of us who've been sick before know all too well how the process works: One of the first things the body does is remove the desire to eat. Once this is taken care of, the body can commence to repair and heal itself.

Nourishment Is Needed

Nature in its wisdom, however, placed a discretionary mechanism within each body system that dictates that *some* form of nourishment continue to be consumed, although in very small amounts and of a very selective quality. Ailing humans get unusual food cravings—

some of them quite weird—that they can respond to by either requesting or getting the items their bodies want.

But this isn't so easy for animals to do. We haven't as yet fully mastered an understanding of a cat's incessant meowing or a dog's endless barking (although some animal psychologists and psychics would like to have us believe otherwise). So what they may want can't be effectively communicated to their owners (dumb us!) as they might like to do. They are fairly limited in procuring what they feel is good for them. I had a sick dog eat lawn grass one time and a not-so-well cat chew flower petals on another occasion.

Getting Rover and Kitty to Eat Again

It may sound trite to some, but getting a sick *animal* to eat something that will do its body good may prove to be more difficult than getting a misbehaving child to eat his or her spinach. Sick animals are not only fussy and obstinate in such circumstances, but they have lost the desire for food. Therefore, some creativity and imagination is needed in order to come up with things that will find definite appeal to their senses of smell, taste, and sight (in that order).

It's real simple to figure out and almost a "no-brainer." Dogs prefer beef (or anything closely resembling it), while cats lean toward anything fishy in nature. Between them they also find pleasure in dining on chicken, turkey, or lamb periodically. Therefore, it makes perfect sense to use any of these items or substitutes that smell and taste like them to entice a sick animal to start eating again.

It is easier for an ailing dog or cat to lap up something with its tongue than to chew. Chewing requires energy that the poor suffering creature may barely have enough of; therefore, whatever is to be served should be in the form of a puree.

The following recipe serves a dual purpose: It can be used for a dog or cat, depending, of course, on which selection of protein is made by the owner. It is versatile enough in nature that other things not listed in the ingredients can be combined or recombined at one's discretion and leisure.

MULTIPURPOSE PET PUREE

1/2 cup raw organic liver (cat or dog)

or

1/2 cup cubed steak (dog) or 1/2 cup fresh, deboned fish (cat)

1 teaspoon Pines barley grass

1/2 teaspoon liquid Kyolic aged-garlic extract

5 drops liquid ConcenTrace

1/2 cup goat's milk (packaged or fresh)

1/2 cup cooked quinoa (cereal grain from South America)

2 raw, organic eggs

Mix everything together in the order given in a blender or food processor. Feed only one-half to three-quarters cup of this mixture each day to a sick animal; slightly increase these amounts proportionately for a larger animal. Refrigerate the rest.

If the animal sniffs the food but doesn't appear to be eating any of it, then put on a glove and scoop up small gobs of this puree on a finger. With the other hand, gently pry the mouth apart. Then quickly smear the puree in the other hand on the roof of the pet's mouth, just behind its front teeth. An animal, no matter how sick, will generally swallow the mixture rather than attempt to spit it out. Take your time in doing this and above all, *don't hurry* this procedure. A sick animal needs time to absorb this food, even in small amounts. Insert another gob a minute later, and so forth. Don't give too much; it's better to feed smaller amounts more often than larger ones infrequently.

If this doesn't work, switch to another method. Thin the recipe down with a little more goat's milk and insert it in a turkey baster or plastic syringe (minus the needle). Most veterinarians should be willing to provide you with one at a nominal fee. Feed a sick animal small amounts about every four hours. Since neither procedure is very conducive to the finicky nature of a cat (and its claws), it would be well for the animal to be wrapped up in an old bath towel before finger- or tube-feeding commences.

If the owner feels that organic raw-meat puree is inappropriate for a sick animal to have, then beef, chicken, or fish bouillon cubes may be used instead to create the flavor and smell of the real things. One bouillon cube can be dissolved in a little hot water and then mixed in with the rest of the foregoing ingredients.

Watch for Dehydration

A sick animal will always be in a state of dehydration. Therefore, it is extremely important to keep a fresh supply of water in its dish at all times. *Do not use tap water.* Instead rely on spring, mineral, or distilled water. Giving a sick animal some *cool* peppermint tea in lieu of water may be even better sometimes. Not only will the tea take care of the dehydration problem, but it will also improve the animal's digestive tract considerably as well as promote an appetite.

Water or tea can also be inserted into an animal's rectum with satisfying results. Use a small rubber syringe or enema bag with a nozzle. Administer the enema over a five-minute period. Lubricate the end with olive oil. Have a family member or friend place the animal in a sink or tub and hold it gently. Be gentle and consistent with the pressure while administering the fluid so it doesn't leak out of the colon. If the liquid refuses to go in, there may be a bowel impactment, in which case the syringe or nozzle will need to be reinserted at a slightly different angle. Generally a bowel evacuation will follow in just a couple of minutes. A sick animal needs such an enema only once a day for a couple of days and no more after that.

If the animal has suffered fluid loss through vomiting or diarrhea, it will be necessary to reintroduce minerals into its system. The best way of doing this is through an enema. Add eight drops of liquid ConcenTrace or Inland Sea Water to the enema for a smaller animal; double or triple this amount for a larger one. (See Product Appendix under Trace Minerals Research for additional information.)

Give Encouragement

A sick animal, like a child or an adult, prefers warmth and attention. A great deal of positive encouragement can be given if the owner will take the time to speak soothing words and frequently rub or brush the animal's coat. Animal instincts are amazingly sharp, and even when sick a cat or dog can still pick up what its owner is thinking or feeling.

Tone of voice and body gestures are dead giveaways. Emotional vibrations from the heart, while usually undetected by humans, are easily discerned by the innate intuition an animal possesses. An owner's attitude, believe it or not, has a lot to do with how a sick animal feels and whether or not it intends to eat.

Consult other entries in the text for additional recipes: Distemper and Feline Leukemia are just two of these.

ANXIETY

A Traveler's Worst Nightmare

Animals can suffer from some of the same types of anxiety that their owners do when exposed to extremely traumatic conditions. The following true story was related to me by a couple at a dog show some time ago. It is related here just as they told it to me, but their names are withheld at their request out of respect for their privacy.

"My husband and I reside in Oregon. We took our prize German shepherd Hunter to a dog show in San Francisco in May 1997. Baggage handlers at the United Airlines terminal there were careless in how they handled our dog's kennel. The door somehow became unlatched allowing our dog to wander off.

"We became frantic after being informed of his escape. The airline official who broke this bad news to us seemed indifferent to the situation and flippantly remarked, 'Oh, it's *only* a dog, for Pete's sakes!' My husband rented a car and we drove around San Francisco International Airport for almost an hour before we found our poor Hunter. Our nine-month-old show dog was lying on the tarmac, whimpering and plumb scared out of his wits. We judged the distance to have been about two miles from where he first got loose."

Calming a Distraught Pooch

"We took him with us to our hotel room. My husband went to a health-food store and bought a box of chamomile tea. I ordered a pitcher of hot water, two cups, and a small bowl to be delivered to our room. I took six tea bags and laid them into the bowl. I poured one cup of water over them and let them soak in it for about 15 minutes. I removed the tea bags and coaxed Hunter into lapping it up. At first he hesitated doing so. But after rubbing his head and neck, kissing him and telling him what a good dog he was, he finally was persuaded to drink the tea. It took about 20 minutes before he finished it, though.

"I made some more tea for my husband and me. I used three tea bags per cup of water, figuring that our nervous systems needed the extra strength. We slowly sipped it and were amazed by how well it relaxed us. Our dog also appeared to be a lot calmer than before. We got ready for that evening's show and groomed Hunter for the occasion. He behaved as if nothing had ever occurred and took second prize.

"About four months after this, we received a check for $610 and a written apology from United Airlines for what had happened. While we appreciated the gesture very much, we don't ever intend flying that airline again, at least not with our dog in tow."

ARTHRITIS

More Common in Dogs

Arthritis is more frequently seen in dogs than in cats, as any veterinarian will tell you. The onset of this inflammatory joint disease is due to immune-mediated causes. Usually chronic infections and immunologic disorders such as systemic lupus erythematosus are the mechanisms that trigger the immune system into actions that simply won't shut off once the main problems have been adequately addressed.

Bone disease often accompanies arthritis. Hip dysplasia is quite common in larger canines because of their extra weight. When the hip sockets of such dogs become malformed due to calcium deposits and severe inflammation, there is a further breakdown of the hips. From the animal's perspective, this can be an excruciating experience.

Both arthritis and hip dysplasia can occur at any age in both sexes of canines. However, the majority of cases are generally seen in dogs between two-and-a-half and four-and-a-half years of age. An interesting phenomenon I've noticed over the years is that large breeds (German shepherds, Doberman pinschers), sporting breeds (collies, spaniels, golden retrievers, pointers), and toy breeds (terriers, poodles) are more susceptible to these diseases than are mongrels of mixed breeds. Shepherds, in particular, suffer a great deal from both problems, followed by huskies.

Prevention Is the Key

Arthritis and hip dysplasia could be prevented if better care were taken by owners in regard to what they fed their bitches during pregnancy. Commercial dog foods are notorious for not supplying enough well-rounded nutrients for the proper skeletal and tissue formations of unborn pups. As a result, many animals are born with a genetic predisposition for such diseases when they become a little older.

The bitch should be fed a diet that includes raw, organic foods. These can be equally divided between meat and vegetables and herbs, just as long as they are rich in calcium, magnesium, potassium, phosphorus, boron, and silicon. Making a soup or stew from leftover chicken or turkey parts in which is included plenty of finely cut carrots, beets, celery, and parsnips is one way to ensure that your pregnant female dog is getting sufficient minerals. Adding a couple of empty eggshells increases the calcium content even more.

Another handy method is to give her lots of fresh salads. You read it right the first time—salads for your dog. In this case, though, you would want to finely grate the carrots, beets, and celery and then work in some minced raw chicken or turkey giblets. You can also use finely chopped beef parts for this, too—liver, heart, tongue, and brain work well here. And, for extra mineral boost, try adding some powdered alfalfa (no more than one-half teaspoon).

A liquid ionic mineral product from the Great Salt Lake is ideal to add to a pregnant bitch's drinking water on a daily basis. About 15 drops of ConcenTrace is adequate. (See the Product Appendix under Trace Minerals Research for more information.)

If you feed your female canine a good diet, her pups will grow up to become healthy and strong dogs with very little chance of ever incurring arthritis or hip dysplasia. But you must start to feed the mother natural food and get away from the commercial junk if you hope to break the vicious cycle of arthritis and bone disease that many dogs will eventually come down with due to the carelessness and stupidity of their owners.

Shark Cartilage Saved a Guide Dog from Arthritis

From 1996 to 1997 I served as the president of the downtown Salt Lake City Lions Club. As a community-service club, the Lions have been recognized for decades for their work with the blind, thanks to the challenge that Helen Keller gave them at one of their first conventions a long time ago. During the state convention of Utah Lions held at the Utah Valley Community College in Orem, I met a sight-impaired man who had come to give our convention delegates a motivational speech on turning your handicaps into strengths.

The man's first name was Teddy. We sat together during lunch. I complimented him on his fine talk and the beautiful-looking German shepherd beside him. He informed me the dog's name was Isak. Then he told me an incredible tale of how he had cured this animal of arthritis.

The dog's condition came to his attention one day on a city bus when a passenger remarked to him that his animal seemed to be dragging one of his hind feet a bit. Teddy had a friend take him and dog to a local vet, who diagnosed the condition as arthritis and recommended a popular drug (Adequan) for it. But Teddy decided to try something natural first before resorting to chemical agents for the animal he had become so attached to.

One day while listening to the radio at home, he heard an advertisement for shark cartilage. He asked a friend to buy him some at a nearby health-food store and commenced giving it to Isak. "I sprinkled one teaspoonful of the powder over his dog food every day," Teddy confided. "Within a couple of weeks, friends and relatives around me began noticing a difference in the way my dog walked. I even felt around his hip and the leg that had been troubling him and could tell it was much straighter and stronger than it had been before. I've kept him on the stuff ever since."

Her Pooch Got Relief the Herbal Way

Millie is a secretary for an insurance-claims adjuster in Toledo, Ohio. She has a little Pekingese called Sniffles. "I gave him this name," she said with a laugh, "because he's always going like this." She then demonstrated for me with a few brief snorts of her own nose what her pooch frequently does. "He doesn't have an allergy. I just think he does it more out of a nervous habit than anything else, especially when people are around. They seem to make him more nervous then."

When Sniffles was diagnosed as having idopathic polyarthritis, she turned to herbs for the solution. "I bought some liquid herbal extracts that were free of alcohol at my health-food store and started giving him these," she said with pride while picking up the dog and giving him a big hug.

The program Millie put her pet on consisted of the following herbal regimen:

Yellow Root	15 drops orally	Early A.M.
Yucca	10 drops orally	Early A.M. Middle P.M.
Vegetal Liquid Liquid Silica (Horsetail)	10 drops in the animal's food	Once daily
Capsaicin Cream (Cayenne Pepper)	Gently massaged through fur onto the skin in a circular motion*	Done several times daily

*CAUTION: Start with a little bit on a small area to begin with and check the site after four hours for adverse reaction such as skin irritation.

After several months on this program, Sniffles was able to maneuver about more easily than before. "Just look at him now," Millie beamed with delight as she held up a bone-shaped doggie treat. Her Pekingese dashed over and began dancing around in a circle with his head arched back waiting to snap it up. "See how quickly he moves," she bragged.

If she hadn't told me of the animal's prior condition, I would never have guessed it once was stricken with arthritis. It is stories such as these from real pet owners that convinced me a long time ago of the value of natural remedies such as herbs in the treatment of many pet health problems. (See the Product Appendix under Nature's Answer for obtaining the herbal extracts mentioned here.)

Something Fishy for Poochy

If you have been led to believe all these years that fish is only for pussycats, then think again: It's also a highly desirable food remedy for treating arthritis in dogs. This can be done one of several ways, but they all involve giving your motion-limited canine shark. That's right, shark as in the monster movie *Jaws*. Great whites and other shark species that give smaller fish perpetual aquatic nightmares carry within their bodies a couple of natural substances that make wonderful antiarthritic remedies.

First there is the much-touted shark cartilage that has gotten tons of global acclaim not only for preventing but also for treating cancer in animals and humans. Further down inside these awesome eating machines may be found their liver oil, which is loaded with compounds called alkylglycerols. When taken and absorbed into an arthritic body, movement becomes considerably easier as pain, joint inflammation, and stiffness gradually subside.

Small dogs should get two capsules per day, while larger ones can handle twice this amount. It is a good idea to give the capsules separate from a meal or just prior to feeding time. (See the Product Appendix under Scandinavian Naturals for a shark supplement that will really take a bite out of your pet's physical misery.)

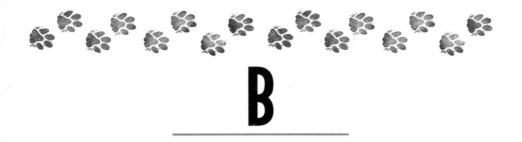

B

BAD BREATH

Tricks for Reducing Animal Halitosis

The expression "dog breath" can apply both to canines as well as to many of their owners. Believe it or not, the solutions for correcting both are quite similar. Over the years I've taken my recommendations for people and have slightly readapted them for application to household pets. By following these procedures for your animal companion, as well as for yourself, the problem of bad breath for both should disappear within a short time.

1. Reduce excess meat intake. Too much animal protein in the diet at any time will invariably produce gastrointestinal fermentation, the effects of which will be smelled later on either as gas discharged from the rectum or else as a sour odor coming out of the mouth. Dry dog food is preferable to table scraps for reducing this problem. However, a happy medium can be struck by alternating between both and giving 50 percent of each at *separate* feedings.

2. Incorporate more vegetable matter into the diet. Carrots, beets, parsnips, and red potatoes may be *gradually* worked into a dog's diet. If your canine isn't used to such vegetables, you'll have to do it by degrees until the animal's taste buds become adjusted to accepting these items. Coarsely grating them in raw form or else cutting into bite-size pieces, *slightly cooking* them, and then draining off all liquid before mixing such vegetables with some canned food or the dried kind that requires a little water may be the best options to pursue.

3. Papaya tablets assist in the digestion of food. Papaya tablets are an inexpensive way to help control halitosis, whether it be of human or animal origin. These can be purchased in any health-food store. For a canine, it is a good idea to crush one tablet and then mix in the powder with the dog's chow. The enzymes that are present eventually reach the gut, where they assist in the breakdown of consumed food matter. With this increase of stomach enzymes, there is apt to be less fermentation or gas that could produce flatulence or bad breath.

4. Chlorophyll makes the breath sweeter. A familiar remedy for human halitosis, as mentioned in my *Encyclopedia of Healing Herbs and Spices* (Englewood Cliffs, NJ: Prentice Hall, 1996; p. 364) is chewing a few springs of parsley to help sweeten the breath. This can also be finely minced and included with dog food for similar results. Powdered wheat-grass or barley-grass juice work just as well and are probably easier to use. Sprinkle one-quarter teaspoon over some canned or packaged food that calls for a little water to be added. Stir until well mixed and then give to your dog to eat. The chlorophyll is what produces better-smelling breath.

5. Clean the teeth and tongue periodically. As humans, we are taught to brush, floss, and rinse the mouth regularly in order to maintain good breath. In some countries, such as India, they even teach you how to scrape your tongue with a special device known as a tongue scraper. Indeed, it is quite fashionable there after a meal to retire to the privacy of a bathroom or away from others and spend a few minutes applying some hygienic efforts to your tongue with scrapers made of wood, metal, or plastic. Of course, trying to apply the same techniques to your dog is going to be a tough challenge, to say the least. And since dogs aren't adapted to rinsing and gargling as we are, that leaves only brushing. An old toothbrush will serve the purpose nicely. A small amount of liquid chlorophyll poured into a bowl can be used for repeatedly dipping the brush in. But it usually takes two people to do the job of brushing canine molars effectively—one for holding the animal's mouth open with gloved hands, while the other vigorously brushes both sides of the teeth and even makes a few passes over the tongue. For larger dogs such as Doberman pinschers or German shepherds, the person holding the mouth ajar will need to straddle them close by their forepaws and then lean down. Everything should be done *slowly and gently,* although the entire operation should proceed rather quickly once things get going and should consume no more time than about 30 seconds. My own experience has taught me this is about all the patience that even the most understanding canine is willing to submit to under such strangely perceived conditions.

Barking

Barking Signals a Need for Attention

Animals are like their human counterparts in many ways when it comes to things they need. They will signal in different ways that attention needs to be given them. In cases of danger, where both animal and human lives are in immediate peril, the former are often more sensitive and can detect such things more quickly than we can. Smart owners will, therefore, give heed to the noises or commotions being made and at least investigate the matter more thoroughly. Unwise individuals usually continue to ignore such disturbance until it's too late. Or, if danger isn't lurking, they will retaliate with anger in some way if their animals persist in such aggressive actions.

Parents with newborn babies know too well the familiar cries in the night that keep them awake. Maternal and paternal instincts automatically have them get up out of a restful sleep to check on their squalling offspring and find out what must be done to make baby happy and thereby bring peace to the household once more.

I'm quite sure most of us at one time or another have had to put up with barking dogs in our respective neighborhoods. The first instinct that usually comes to mind is to open the window or go outside and yell in a loud voice, "Ah, shaddup!" The next temptation may be to get a big stick and go over and beat some sense into the stupid mutt. But that usually passes from our minds very quickly due to the legal complications it involves.

But we shouldn't feel despair under such circumstances if we just take a few minutes to collect our thoughts, keep our cool, and

try to see things from the *dog's* point of view. I know this suggestion may sound somewhat goofy, but after hearing me out you'll see
the common-sense value to it. With the exception of prowlers, imminent earthquakes, storms, and, oh yes, roaming cats, there are other
things that can make a dog bark loudly and long.

Insecurity, anxiety, loneliness, grief, or general unhappiness
generally are the other reasons that canines voice themselves in such
irritating crescendos of sound. Little wonder, since dogs seem to
have evolved from tame wolves and wild coyotes and jackals almost
100,000 years ago, according to an article in the June 28, 1997, issue
of *Science News* (151:400–401). Zoologists and other researchers
analyzed DNA from 162 wolves representing 27 populations in
Europe, Asia, and North America. The results were then compared
with DNA from 140 dogs representing 67 breeds around the world,
from the African basenji to the Irish wolfhound. An unmistakable
connection between the two was made. With this evolutionary pattern also came the howling, yipping, or singing common to wolves,
jackals, and coyotes.

Thus came about for dogs their unique and distinctive way of
expressing themselves when in pain or sorrow—barking. Just as the
normally behaved person would never strike a crying baby to
silence him or her, so would an individual not want to hit or yell at
a barking mutt.

Niceness Cures Neuroses

The father of modern psychoanalysis, Sigmund Freud, never bothered to include domesticated animals in his "couch-therapy" recommendations. But kindness and understanding are universal traits and
apply with equal measure to pets as well as to people. Screaming at,
hitting, or throwing something toward a barking dog only escalates
the barking and further intensifies the situation. Granted that the animal may be intimated enough to cease for the moment, but rest
assured the barking will resume before long.

If it's someone else's dog that's making the racket, your options
are limited. You can either speak with the owner the next day about
the problem or else get yourself a good set of earplugs. But if your

own pooch is the culprit, the remedies are fairly easy and quite rewarding.

1. Sit down beside your dog, or if it's small enough, place it in your lap.
2. Gently stroke the animal with your hand; brush its coat.
3. While doing so, engage in a soft conversation with the dog. Conduct it just as you would for a distressed human whom you loved a lot. Obviously, the animal won't be able to understand the exact words you're saying. But the *tones and gestures* will definitely suggest to this frustrated pet that you are someone who certainly loves it a lot.
4. Walking and even playing with a dog under stress will help to take its mind off whatever was annoying it in the first place.
5. Even having your dog sleep in bed with you (good for smaller animals) or else on the floor beside you (preferable for larger-sized species) will contribute to an increase in its own security. As I said before, dogs are no different from us in this respect. And the closer they can be to those to whom they are fondly attached, the better for everyone concerned.

Train Them While They're Young

The old adage "You can't teach an old dog new tricks" seems apropos when it comes to stopping incessant barking. Pups are always much easier to train in this respect. Helping a young dog understand words such as "Quiet" or "Peace" instills at an early age the command to stop barking. Also, giving the pup a rubber bone to chew on or a favorite toy to play with when it commences barking draws an association in the young animal's mind with fun over noisemaking.

Laying the groundwork for minimal barking when the pooch gets older is an investment of time, energy, considerable patience, and lots of love. At the same time, though, the owner must establish in the pup's mind just who is in charge. Young animals, like children, if properly taught correct behavior, will conduct themselves that way as they become older.

Interacting with your animal as often as possible is especially important if you wish to have good relations with it. Even cats, which are highly individualistic and have minds of their own, as well as dogs, which are extremely sociable creatures, can prove to be cooperative when raised in the right kind of environment.

BEHAVIOR PROBLEMS

Inappropriate Adult Responses

Sometimes in life we must see things through an exaggerated perspective in order to fully appreciate their depth and seriousness. What would happen to an adult human being if he or she were to do any of the following activities:

- Jump on another person
- Bite or scratch someone else without provocation
- Chase or attack another person for no reason
- Make excessive noise in the house or neighborhood
- Use someone's front lawn or public sidewalk as a toilet
- Dig a hole in the neighbor's backyard
- Trespass on private property without permission

I called the Salt Lake City Police Department and spoke with Detective "John Doe" in the Investigations Division. (Police policy doesn't allow the names of any officers to be used in an interview situation without prior authorization from the chief of police himself; hence the use of John Doe here.) I asked him what might be the charge for each of the preceding misbehaviors if he or one of his fellow detectives were investigating the matter. Here is what he told me:

- Jumping on someone else would be considered an assault.
- Biting or scratching would be written up as mayhem.

- Attacking someone else would be an aggravated assault.
- Excessive noise-making is a simple disorderly-conduct charge.
- Public urination/defecation is plain lewdness.
- Digging in your neighbor's yard is criminal mischief.
- Trespassing is just that—trespassing!

Officer Doe informed me that for some of these charges, the investigating officer would just write a ticket. But in more severe cases he would be apt to arrest the offender on the spot and transport the individual to the city jail. "A lot of what the officer would do," my informant said, "depends on the extreme nature and seriousness of the misbehavior involved."

Common Animal Misbehaviors

Common sense tells us that any responsible person isn't going to behave in any of those inappropriate ways. But, believe it or not, that responsible person's dog or cat is likely to do one or several of those things on a pretty regular basis without any fear of being ticketed or going to the animal shelter. What's even more galling is that a fair number of pet owners, when presented with the evidence of such misbehavior, will shrug it off and casually remark, "Well, dogs will be dogs" or "What else did you expect; that's a cat's nature, for heaven's sakes."

While we can't ever expect our household animals to be as law-abiding and thoughtful as we are in every situation, we do understand that there is an *implied* obligation on our parts to at least teach them good behavior or control them or clean up their messes. This is part of what constitutes being a good citizen of the community. Besides obeying a number of municipality laws such as driving carefully, respecting others, and not littering, there are also on the books of many cities local ordinances governing the actions of people's pets. These must be taken more seriously by owners, and greater efforts must be made to obey them, too, just as we would obey those statutes governing our own activities.

Jumping Is a Definite No-No

How often do we find situations in which people who are visiting friends and relatives suddenly find themselves being pawed by the other's medium-sized or large dog? If dressy clothing is worn, it can become muddied or torn in the process. Also, older folks and younger children often become frightened by such unexpected canine enthusiasm. A delicate situation is then created between both parties by such doggie misbehavior. The recipients may be hesitant to say anything for fear of offending the pet owners. After all, friendships and family ties may be at stake here, and who wants to risk verbally injuring or possibly insulting someone else for whom deep feelings and cherished ties have been longheld?

If an overfriendly mutt heads your way in leaps and bounds and intends to paw you, don't become upset. Sudden hostile human reactions can confuse an otherwise loving animal. Turn to one side, bow your head slightly, and keep your hands down. But raise one hand slightly, fold in the thumb and other fingers, leaving only the second "pointer" finger sticking out. Then in a gentle but firm voice say, "No! No! No!" while at the same time making short, downward-chopping motions with your pointer finger. Stand your ground, show no fear or anxiety, and be firm but loving.

For a pet owner the solution is simple—it's spelled out in the form of a l-e-a-s-h. If an owner knows that his or her dog is a jumper, then that person has an obligation to restrain such canine enthusiasm by keeping the dog properly leashed or fenced in. That way neither clothes nor personal dignity nor relationships are ruined.

What to Do About Unprovoked Biting or Scratching

Some incidents of biting or scratching by a household pet can be avoided with a little common sense. Young children are apt to tease an animal by pulling on its ears (which are extremely sensitive), rubbing its fur the wrong way, tugging the tail (also very sensitive), chasing and cornering it, playfully wrestling with it (if a larger animal), picking it up against its will (a small dog or a cat), and other equally silly antics. Dogs seem to have a much greater tolerance level for *some* of this foolishness, but cats definitely do not. They burn a much shorter fuse and can get impatient very quickly; when that happens look out for a quick retaliatory response to put an end to such nonsense.

Sometimes overdoing a good thing can induce a negative action from a household pet. Consider what happened to an elderly lady named Mrs. Blake who lived on Cape Cod, Massachusetts. As animal psychologist Dr. Nicholas Dodman reported in *The Cat Who Cried for Help* (New York: Bantam Books, 1997; pp. 66-68), she called his "behavior hotline seeking advice about her six-year-old white split-eyed cat" named Casper. He discovered that this neutered male "would often bite her while she was petting him." After considerable inquiry, he diagnosed the problem as "petting-induced aggression." He advised her to read the obvious warning signals when Casper felt he had enough physical attention and wanted her to quit: tail-twitching at the tip, sideways glances, sudden and constant pupil enlargement or diminishment, and frequent head tilts. He told her to keep the petting sessions brief and make them less often than usual.

In a few weeks Mrs. Blake reported on how she and her tabby were getting along. "Apparently Casper had not bitten her at all while being petted because she had effectively rationed his pettings and had learned to spot the telltale premonitory signs during what were not less frequent petting bouts," he wrote.

Other factors, however, that may induce unprovoked biting or scratching from an otherwise usually friendly animal sometimes cannot be helped. When my staff and I relocated our research center to the floor below us in the building we've been in for many years, we could no longer have the pleasure of our office cat's company. I had to make other arrangements for Jake. I thought I had found a nice home for him in the small south-central Utah community of Gunnison with a widow and her 20-year-old son, both of whom loved cats very much. But scarcely a week had passed when I received a distressing phone call from the lady, who had to be rushed to the emergency ward of the local hospital to have a nasty gash in her upper forearm closed, where my cat had slashed her with his claws. In the meantime, Jake had been taken to the local animal shelter and was destined for Kingdom Come had I not driven down and bailed him out of his temporary prison.

I came to learn how the unexpected attack happened. This woman's *other* cat (that I never knew about), which ordinarily stayed outside, decided to wander into her house one day. Jake and the other feline promptly got into a cat fight of major proportions. The woman unwisely tried to separate them and in the process got badly mauled by my animal.

Not wanting this to happen again for fear of risking a lawsuit, I made the tough decision to take my cat to our family ranch in the southern Utah wilderness, where I turned him loose. He went for a number of months without any ranch hand and stayed in the upper hay loft of our big barn during that period of time. His natural hunting instincts took over and he survived (though barely) on pack rat, field mice, occasional squirrels, and even a scorpion or two. For water he drank out of the nearby creek or ate snow in the winter time.

As I review Jake's remarkable nine lives, I can see what brought on this Dr. Jekyll–Mr. Hyde transformation. Jake's original world of the office and staff he knew and loved had suddenly been turned upside down. His heretofore fairly tranquil existence had just become violently disrupted. The cat I knew who used to love lying across the back top of my padded office chair as I sat and typed in the evening and who would periodically caress me with his head, had suddenly changed into a very hostile animal.

From that one sad experience I've learned several things. First, cats are more subject to the stress of moving or relocation than dogs are. Second, one-owner cats find it much more difficult to readjust to someone else than canines do. Third, even careful placement in a loving environment around other kind people may not always satisfy a feline used to someone else from kittenhood. Fourth, I've vowed to *never again* get another kitten unless I'm absolutely sure I can keep it for the rest of its natural life.

There are some logical steps to take, however, to curb senseless biting and clawing in your pet. Make or buy a scratching post on which your pussy can stretch and exercise its claws. A square 4x4 post that is about 18 inches high and securely mounted on a wide, heavy plywood-board base to which has been affixed a carpet remnant of tight weave makes a dandy post that every cat in the neighborhood would envy. Periodically soak small spots of the carpet with a little catnip oil or catnip tincture. Felines will find it irresistible. Also, administering small doses of St. John's Wort tincture or fluid extract (no more than eight drops at a time) helps to control unnecessary provocation. Be sure, though, that the liquid solution you use is *alcohol-free*.

Manifested Aggression

In his other book, *The Dog Who Loved Too Much* (New York: Bantam Books, 1997), Dr. Dodman addresses some of the issues that might make a normally friendly dog become mean and ill-tempered. Fear or anger are the main factors for bringing about these changes. An animal "is frightened by loud noises" or can "suffer from separation anxiety." Cruel treatment or hostile emotions can easily invoke anger in a generally peaceable and playful canine. Dr. Dodman makes a good point of owner behavior inducing insecure feelings in some dogs: "Owners can unwittingly escalate the fearful response [by acting] nervously themselves, which simply compounds the dog's fear. Owners who tense up . . . send a message to the dog that there is trouble ahead . . . " Also, the size of a canine can play a role in its level or aggression: "Large dogs may be more intimidating and may advance more quickly through the ranks of the shy sharp biters." To this, however, I would like to add that smaller sizes such as terriers or Chihuahuas can be equally pesky in their own right: They are unforgiving heel nippers and ankle biters.

Dr. Dodman has a standard approach for such hostile reactions, which he terms "desensitization." He claims that it "is central to [the] treatment" of an aggressive animal. The basic elements of the remarkable therapy are these:

1. Very slowly and gradually introduce the animal to whatever may frighten it (for example, vacuum cleaner, lawn mower, automobile, children, other pets, and so forth). With each level of introduction, the *distance* between such things and the nervous pet (which started out considerable) become less and less until it can feel reasonably comfortable being near them. And with each attempt at this, always be sure that "the dog is richly rewarded with food treats, praise, and petting for remaining calm when confronted" with the object or person at varying distances.

2. If the animal is permitted to be indoors, then provide it with some sort of "safe haven" into which it can crawl for security. This animal den "should be made welcoming by putting a blanket, toys, and perhaps food treats inside." Such a den needn't be elaborate, an old crate will do just fine, although cats may prefer a cardboard box (empty orange or apple box) or basket. This haven should be off-limits to kids and away from general household noise such as radio or television.

3. Employ a tape recorder as part of the desensitization process. Playing disturbing sounds at low-intensity around the animal may allow it to grow accustomed to them even when the objects that generate these sounds aren't around or in use at the time.

4. Incorporate a leash or halter when *slowly* reintroducing an animal to people it may not like. Don't force the issue; let the animal take its own time through sniffing and eyeballing the individual (from a safe distance, of course, while you maintain a firm grip on the leash) to determine if it wants to be friendly or not.

5. Be generous with your affection: pat the animal's head, stroke its coat, and even hug it to give reassurance that it is loved and deeply appreciated. But, likewise, don't overdo a good thing either. Positive reinforcement is just fine, but as with children, an excessive amount can make a pet spoiled rotten. A sensible balance must be kept between the owner's firmness and his or her loving kindness. You never want to be so dominant as to instill boss-like fear, but at the same time you must be definite on certain points so the animal will come to respect you and know who is in control.

6. Exercise is another part of this counterconditioning. A dog should have a least "twenty to thirty minutes of aerobic exercise" every day. And though Dr. Dodman doesn't mention it in either of his two books, I would like to mention *travel* here. Taking a dog or cat on frequent short trips—better use a small carry-all for kitty—around town can do wonders for neurotic pets. I discovered this quite by accident some years ago while working with a doctor who treated disturbed children under

the age of 12. I was amazed at how much they calmed down whenever he and some of his staff would take them around town in the clinic van. The difference it made was like night and day; they were more calm while out sightseeing. I began recommending this to a number of owners with agitated pets. The "trip therapy," as I dubbed it, worked well: Both dogs and (to a lesser extent) cats seemed to enjoy themselves immensely and "forgot" the reasons for their previous aggressions.

Certain physical ailments can produce untoward aggression. Dr. Dodman lists these in *The Cat Who Cried for Help*: "partial seizures, thiamine deficiency, sugar diabetes, and advanced hepatic or renal disease." (Look under Diabetes, Epilepsy, Kidney Stones, and Liver Problems, for additional data on resolving these problems naturally.) He believes that "an all-fish diet" induces a vitamin B-1 deficiency in cats that could bring out unanticipated hostilities. Administering a good B-complex formula to your pet should clear this up. Just crush one tablet (cats) or two (dogs) into powder before mixing in with the animal's food. The addition of one-half teaspoon (cats) to one tablespoon (dogs) of brewer's-yeast powder in the food dish also resolves any B deficiencies that may exist.

The periodic washing and drying of an animal is bound to bring out the worst in some of them. Dogs as a rule don't mind being bathed; in fact, they actually like to be squirted with a hose and find it rather amusing. Not so with cats, however; most cats despise water immersion with a passion and will fight like hell to get out of it. Take my word for it—I learned the hard way and had the scratches to prove it! However, a former part-time staff member (a high-school kid named Matt) could bathe Jake without the cat going berserk. So to him was assigned this periodic task. I watched with amazement how he did it with nary a scratch, hiss, or bite. He used lukewarm water (not very much either) and slowly introduced the cat to that until it had become somewhat accepting of it. All the while he carried on a one-sided conversation with Jake, speaking in low, soft, soothing tones to him. It took him *twice* as long to bathe Jake as it did for me, but he certainly wasn't scratched or bitten as I often was. When his employment ended, I came up with another plan. I spent part of one day going through the business Yellow Pages of our local telephone directory until I found a professional grooming service that took care of cats, but *without* anesthetizing them first. I learned to my astonishment that anesthetizing is a fairly common procedure for many animal groomers who do cats—it simplifies things and greatly reduces the risk of personal injury, but at obvious cost to feline health. So before you entrust your cat to a grooming agency, be sure to ask them if they put kitty into la-la land with drugs before bathing it. If they do, look around for someone who doesn't. In the event you can't find such a service, then do it yourself.

Neighborhood Animal Symphonies

There is nothing more annoying than a barking dog or a yowling cat when you're trying to think, relax, or sleep. Just ask someone who's had that happen to him or her if you haven't experienced the situation firsthand yourself. Canine yapping is probably the biggest complaint pet owners hear from annoyed neighbors. And cats in heat, cats doing a circular face-off opposite one another or else actually fighting can produce some of the most eerie sounds imaginable; and they get only spookier in the dark.

When someone comes to your house you obviously want your dog to detect it before you do and start barking. But the dog also needs to know when to be still after being reassured that things are okay. Training for this should ideally begin when it is a mere puppy; but not fully matured dogs can also be coached. It is more difficult with older canines, however. The groundwork for this needs to be laid with considerable time, patience, and love. The puppy or older dog needs to understand the meaning of the word "quiet." For myself, I've always preferred the word "peace" instead; it has one-syllable and sounds more pleasing to the ear. It also seems easier for canine comprehension. Repeated use of the word and constant reward for following this instruction will pay off in big dividends. But be sure to differentiate when barking is appropriate and when it isn't; otherwise you might wind up with a mute animal silently watching a thief burglarize your premises.

Getting a cat to stop its constant meowing is another matter. Cats have a mind of their own, as any cat owner should know. An investigation into the reason for such feline racket is warranted. The animal may be injured, sick, or lonely. Maybe all it needs is a little attention, food, exercise, or brushing. When my office cat Jake would occasionally meow for a few minutes, one of my staff or I would check the matter and try to determine the cause for it. More often than not, it was one of the reasons just given for which so much noise was being made.

Inappropriate Elimination

Animals, just as humans, must be potty-trained, and it begins when they are very young. Kittens need to learn where their litter box is and to use it consistently. If they relieve themselves anywhere else, they must be properly taught that this is unacceptable behavior. There are a number of ways to do this. One of the most successful has been to pick up or wipe up the mess with a paper towel and carry it, together with the kitten, and place both in the litter box side by side. The offensive material can then be brought close to the kitten's nose, while gently holding its tiny head with two fingers. The matter is then laid back down on top of the litter material and the kitten's attention is focused to both at once by pointing and repeatedly saying, "Here, Here" or "Yes, Yes."

A variation on the same theme is to point to the mess on the floor before cleaning it up and holding the kitten's head quite close to it, gently saying over and over again, "No, No, No, No," and then soaking a cotton ball in a little vinegar and lightly dabbing it on the end of the kitty's nose. A few times of this treatment and its fertile feline brain will quickly draw an association between messy floors or carpeting and bad smells. Positive reinforcement comes by rubbing a catnip mouse or herbal sachet filled with mint against its nose while it is sitting in the litter box with its cleaned-up bodily wastes. The vinegar-on-nose treatment also works for young puppies.

For older cats who periodically insist on dumping somewhere outside their litter boxes, owners must assume more of a feline attitude. That is, they must think something like their cats would. Generally, this kind of unacceptable behavior from an older cat who should know better might be due to unhappiness in its environment.

"It's a cat's way of expressing agitation, not a personal message to you," writes Richard H. Pitcairn, DVM in his book, *Dr. Pitcairn's Complete Guide to Natural Health for Dogs & Cats* (Emmaus, PA: Rodale Press, Inc., 1995; p. 163). This could mean that "the litter box is not clean enough or the particular litter that's used is not to their liking." Occasionally, it can be something as simple as your relocating the litter box from your cat's favorite place to one that is less preferred, in its estimation.

A male is sometimes apt to spray or "mark" its territory if another pet or new person (newborn infant) enters the household or if the owner moves into new surroundings with which the cat may be totally unfamiliar. "Inappropriate elimination may also signal chronic health problems such as allergies," Dr. Pitcairn writes.

In a rather thought-provoking chapter entitled, "To Pee or Not to Pee" in his book *The Dog Who Loved Too Much,* animal therapist Dr. Nicholas Dodman offers some curious insights into the canine psychology possibly lurking behind every elimination. For example, one amazing thought of Dr. Dodman's: "The deposition of urine and feces is also a means of visual and olfactory communication"— sort of a doggie equivalent of "Kilroy was here." Such canine calling cards are really biological scent markers known as pheromones. By smelling its own waste materials for a few seconds, the dog gets a heightened sense of its own well-being and self-importance. And sniffing the doo-doo of other mutts gives the animal a better understanding of their particular biochemical makeup. In a word, it's pretty much a hormonal thing between canines.

Dogs are inherently clean creatures and will usually avoid defecating or urinating in areas generally designated for dining, sleeping, and romping. This fastidiousness with their toiletry is believed to have evolved tens of thousands of years ago when humans first domesticated wolves as cave pets for pleasure, utility, and protection. If a dog soils in the house, it usually means one of two things: Either its owner forgot to take it outside or the animal is emotionally frustrated over something.

A good rule of thumb to remember is that a puppy can hold its urine for the number of hours that corresponds to its age in months plus one. By the time a dog has reached maturity, however, it can go up to ten hours without having to trot outside to urinate. But if the canine is being fed a high fiber diet (see Diet Tips), then it stands to reason it will have to defecate much sooner than otherwise.

It has been claimed by some old-timers that if you rub a puppy's nose in its own mess or whack it with a newspaper on the behind *and* do the other that you will soon correct it of its house-soiling ways. This may be true, but it also runs the risk of engendering fear in the young animal as well. I prefer the vinegar dab-on-the-nose treatment followed with several sharp but definite "No's" to get the point across

A slight variation on this method is to lay the forefinger somewhat hard across the dog's snout, while firmly saying "No" a number of times. This does away with the vinegar dabbing but usually gets the same results.

When a responsible pet owner is out walking his or her dog, the person doesn't allow the dog to answer the call of nature wherever it feels like it. Public and private properties should be respected at all times. And in the event a messing incident accidentally happens on such premises, then the owner is obligated to clean the mess then and there. Walking a dog on a leash can prevent this from happening most of the time.

Whoever Heard of an Animal Reading a Sign?

Animals may be smart and have intuitive powers far beyond our own, but we can at least read and decipher the meaning of posted signs, where they cannot. Thus, a "No Trespassing" sign means just that. But for the average dog, that means *nothing*. It will trot over, crawl through, or run across private or public property, never knowing such action is forbidden. That duty is left up to the owner, who needs to keep the dog leashed or properly fenced in. This way no backyards get dug up or front lawns get pooped on. The neighbors remain . . . well, neighborly.

But trying to get a cat not to do this is to ask for the impossible. Felines are single-minded when it comes to doing what they want to do. They are used to getting their own way, and their adventuresome spirits lead wherever curiosity and instinct take them. A reasonable solution is to raise a cat kept indoors most of the time. That way there are virtually no outside distractions to tempt it.

Frequent Licking

Animals prefer to lick themselves periodically. Most of it is usually for grooming purposes, but sometimes it can help heal an external injury. Saliva is an amazing substance and contains many interesting compounds. Among them is one called epidermal or nerve-growth factor (EGF or NGF). This has the capability of promoting more rapid wound healing or tissue reunification.

Cats lick themselves more often than most other animals do. It is their way of staying clean. People who are allergic to cats (as I have been prone to be in times past) have developed a hypersensitivity to the *dried* saliva that sticks to the animal's hair. This and the dander it produces is what makes many people sneeze and experience watering and itching of the eyes at the same time. Generally speaking, it's okay for cats to lick themselves a lot; it's what comes naturally to them and what they seem to enjoy doing.

But there are limits to how often a dog may lick a certain portion of its body, say a forelimb or a hind limb or chest if it's lying down. When a canine becomes utterly bored or really stressed over something, it will start licking a favorite spot to relieve this boredom or for comfort. In time this behavior can become so ingrained that it is performed at any time, even when boredom or stress do not exist.

Giving a dog some fluid extract of St. John's Wort (10-20 drops daily) or several capsules (3) of valerian root may help to prevent the continuation of this problem. Making sure the animal is happy and never left alone for very long are of equal consideration here. Providing an ample number of chewable toys is another way of alleviating this situation.

So Human an Animal

Scientists engaged in the study of certain species of animals around the world have reported seeing a surprising number of human characteristics in many of them. This fact prompted one scholar to coin the term, "so human an animal," thereby signifying the uncanny closeness between men and beasts.

In my business of anthropology, I have been engaged in the general physical and social study of human beings. In the process of doing my work, I've had a tendency to wander over to the animal side of things and to study them as well. With the passing of years, this inclination has become more frequent. It is now evident to me that many of the traits that make us good or bad can also be found within animals.

What makes a dog "man's best friend"? Is it not the loyalty and devotion beating within its canine heart? May not the same be found in an elderly couple who've been happily married for 50 years or longer? And how about patience? Wouldn't dogs walk away with the trophy more often for this than we humans would? On the other hand, the killer instincts of a psychotic human parallel the nearly intense emotions of crazed pit bull terriers or fierce boxers. And what about the finicky ways of spoiled children or hard-to-live-with wives? Could not many similarities between them and fussy felines be found?

In conclusion, the real secret to resolving animal behavior problems is to start thinking as they do. Once that has been achieved, just about any solution is possible.

Bladder Problems

Litter-Box Blues

An obsolete medical term, *stranguria,* was once commonly used by many veterinarians to describe bladder difficulties in household pets. Bladder inflammation is more frequently seen in cats than it is in dogs. The lining of the pet's bladder and urethra become inflamed, making urination extremely difficult and painful. The animal must, in effect, physically strain itself in order to evacuate a minimum amount of urine.

Anxious owners will generally rush their poor, suffering pets to their veterinarians where a catheter is inserted to relieve the swelling and permit urine to pass out. Elective surgery is often recommended and consented to by pet owners. But not all vets are knife-and-drug happy; some, in fact, opt to pursue alternative measures that are far less invasive and have virtually no side effects.

Here is a true case shared by one alternative practitioner named Cheryl Schwartz, DVM. A woman named Mylene brought her blond cat decorated with red stripes to Dr. Schwartz's animal clinic. The vet carefully examined Poosha and then asked the owner a series of questions in order to get a better grasp on the animal's medical plight. It seems that for the previous several months the cat had spent much of her time straining and crying at the litter box, unable to urinate more than a few drops before collapsing, frustrated and exhausted, her belly pressed against the cool litter.

The veterinarian watched as the cat attempted to walk. Her slightly bloated abdomen swung tightly as she took a few hesitant steps. Her face was pinched with anxiety and her body was tight with fear. It was obvious to both the owner and doctor that this animal was in a great deal of pain.

Getting Poosha Well with Traditional Chinese Medicine

Dr. Schwartz practices in the San Francisco Bay area and has access to a lot of data concerning traditional Chinese medicine. She has acquainted herself with much of this, believing that it helps in her practice and makes treatments a lot safer for the variety of animals that she sees on a daily basis.

The vet prescribed three Chinese herbs: prunella, atractylodes, and Asiatic plantain. She recommended the liquid extracts that were alcohol-free. In the event Mylene couldn't get these for her pet, she was to mix ten drops of each alcohol-based herbal extract in an ounce of distilled water before dispensing it. An average of one teaspoon daily of these three herbs combined was poured directly down Poosha's throat. (In the event these herbs can't be procured, an alcohol-free liquid herb extract called Bladdex may be obtained from Nature's Answer. See the Product Appendix.)

Another modality that Dr. Schwartz prescribed was simple massage. She noted that "a massage can comfort an animal's tired muscles, relieve pain, and restore flexibility." The massage routine devised by her helped boost Poosha's circulation and strengthen the cat's internal organs. She showed Mylene how to do it on her pet. A light fingertip pressure was applied along the midline of the cat's belly, beginning at the top of her rib-cage and extending every inch down to the pelvis. Mylene was also told to massage the lower belly, using sweeping, circular strokes in a clockwise direction and passing the fingertips along the last three rib case spaces, on both sides of the body. Mylene performed this massage twice a day on her beloved Poosha.

Several months went by before Poosha showed complete recovery from her symptoms. These methods took considerably longer than conventional surgery or drugs would have done. But, at least, they were natural and safe and pain-free. At last report the pussy and her person were both doing extremely well.

Rover Got over His Problem

A construction worker named George has a mixed-breed, medium-sized dog he calls Rover. His dog began experiencing some bladder problems. George's live-in girlfriend works at a local health-food store. She thought some liquid herbal extracts might do the trick. With her boyfriend's permission, she combined 15 drops each of sarsaparilla, red clover, and barberry and gave it to Rover orally twice a day for two weeks. She also fed him a tablespoon of cod-liver oil and one teaspoon of liquid vitamin C every day, too.

Rover soon recovered from his bladder discomforts and was himself again, much to the delight of George and his girlfriend. This made a believer in herbs out of him, and he started using some of them to improve his own health.

BODY ODORS

The World's Most Inscrutable Creature

On the popular PBS educational program *Nature* (with host George Page), a recent edition was devoted exclusively to the mysterious and wonderful world of cats. Among many different cultures worldwide, the cat is considered to be "an inscrutable creature." The cat was worshipped in ancient Egypt and even mummified occasionally.

Cats are solitary creatures except for lions, which are the only members of the huge cat family that move in social circles. The tiger most closely resembles a house cat, being able to skillfully blend in with its natural surroundings. The cheetah is the only cat whose method of hunting closely parallels that of the dog, because it chases its quarry down instead of stalking it like other large cats do.

Cats were believed to be omens of evil and were therefore, routinely destroyed in the Middle Ages. It wasn't until the introduction to the great bubonic plague via the brown rat that cats came to be appreciated for their rodent-hunting skills. It is said that those households that kept a cat close by suffered the least from this Black Death epidemic.

"Cats live in a whole landscape of odors that we are totally unfamiliar with," the program narrator mentioned. Cats assume various body postures according to the type of odors they encounter. A hint of dog in the air immediately puts the cat in a defensive mode of attack, while a scent of catnip reduces a feline to a very relaxed and extremely playful position. When a female cat is in heat she sends out a number of scent signals that attract all of the available male cats that may be in the immediate neighborhood. But she is finicky about which suitor she wants to mate with and will violently repel all those who don't seem to have "the correct odor" that pleases her.

When a cat rubs against some part of your body, it isn't necessarily showing its affection, but, in fact, may actually be marking you with one of its distinctive scents. This is a cat's way of including someone it likes within its territorial domain. In a household where two or more cats are present, each one may, in turn, come up to the individual, sniff the odor from the previous feline and then go about adding its own scent by similarly rubbing up against some part of the person's body.

Cats' Sense of Smell

This hour-long program covered many other fascinating aspects of the cat world, only a few of which have been cited here. But one of the recurring and dominant themes was the importance of odor to a cat. A cat cannot function without it. Scents of all types govern much of the thinking and action of this animal. They help give it a sense of direction and purpose. An odor-free world would be just as cruel to a cat as would declawing, spaying and neutering, tail-docking, or, worse still, denying it the most basic fundamentals of food or water. A bland atmosphere would drive the average cat completely crazy within a short time. It would, most likely, lose its will to live and perish from stifled boredom, if nothing else.

The program made a special point of cautioning any cat owners who may have been watching that odor control of felines should always be kept to an absolute minimum. A pleasant-smelling litter-box is obviously desirable for the respiratory health of human and pet alike; but a clean-scented cat (at least by our standards) isn't always necessary, unless there are plans to display it at a cat show. The use of aerosols to "prettify the air" only confuse cats and aggravate existing human allergies, so what's the point in using them?

Putrefaction Needs Attention

Common sense tells us, though, that whenever putrefaction is present in some form, it requires prompt attention. A cat or dog may have dirty teeth that need to be regularly cleaned, either by a veterinarian or the owner. Sometimes bacteria will breed externally on dirty skin, so the animal will need a bath followed by a diluted white-vinegar or lemon-juice rinse to help kill lingering germs.

Making food available at all times isn't a good idea for several reasons. The food itself can easily spoil or attract insects in warm weather, thereby reducing odor. Also, the smell of food reaching an animal's brain will inspire it to eat more frequently even when hunger desires are satisfied. This overeating can fill the animal's body with excess waste materials that push out through the skin pores as oil and dandruff. This not only looks bad but smells terrible.

Soiling is another common cause of body odor. Diarrhea can soil the back legs. Long-haired pets are apt to get dirtied more frequently by dragging their undercoats through badly kept litter boxes or outside ground deposits. Eye and ear discharges also produce secretions that aren't pleasant.

An owner has the responsibility to attend to such matters and resolve them as quickly as possible by whatever methods seem appropriate. Mixing one teaspoon (cats) to one tablespoon (dogs) of brewer's yeast in the food rations every day will help considerably in reducing natural gland or body odors regularly produced by household pets. Try it and you'll be surprised at how effective this simple solution is.

How ACV Turned One Stinky Dog into a Sweet-Smelling Canine

In September 1998 Dr. Bob and Susan Goldstein celebrated the third anniversary of their monthly publication *Love of Animals*. (See Appendix II for subscription information.) They permitted me to reuse this true story, which appeared in their September 1996 issue.

"Mary Demick, a soft-spoken woman from Galveston Island, Texas, has earned the title of healer. Then so has her dog, Ginger. Mary's story demonstrates the power of pursuing natural health one step at a time, building slowly and effortlessly upon success. Add a steadfast commitment and a degree of patience and you have the recipe for an amazing recovery. For seven years, Mary and her mother Alice, battled Ginger's heartbreaking allergies. 'Mother and I have been through a lot of pain and suffering because of Ginger's suffering,'" Mary says of her mischievous 9-year-old retriever.

"In March [1996], Mary and Alice were nearly panicked because Ginger was miserable, frantically licking bare spots in her coat and giving off a putrid smell. Her recent allergy shot lasted only two weeks before the itching returned. After reading about organic apple cider vinegar [ACV] . . . Mary started adding it to Ginger's drinking water. 'The first thing I noticed about the vinegar was that [Ginger's] smell improved quickly,' she says.

"'I started everything out on a small scale. I didn't want to do anything to upset her stomach.' Eventually, Ginger was eating carrots, celery, cabbage and parsley and taking vitamins.

"Mary wrote to us [later] of [an] experiment [she conducted at home.] 'My mother, Alice Demick, is another miracle of yours! She had endured continuous bladder infections from June 1995 until March 10th. We started putting organic apple cider vinegar in our drinking water March 19th and *no more* bladder infections!'

"Long gone are the days of feeding handfuls of Milk Bones and a chemically reserved pet food. 'You love them so much, but you do so many things unknowingly that are bad. I feel so fortunate that we found this out before she got any older.'

"The best gift of all—Mary is convinced—this happier, healthier Ginger is more able than ever to do her work service as the lifeline for Alice, who [turned 89 in October 1996]. 'When Mother broke her hip, the [hip-replacement] surgery was pretty hard on her and she lost some memory.' But Mary's mother never lost touch with reality when it came to Ginger. Alice's broken hip and pelvis have healed. Now, she plays outside with Ginger several times a day without the aid of a walker. 'I'm sure that my mother wouldn't be here if not for Ginger,' says Mary."

BRUISED PAWS

Tender Footpads

Dogs and cats were endowed with protective footpads to help them lope along in a graceful gait or add more spring to their steps when rapid movements become necessary. Sometimes, in the course of their locomotions, they are prone to getting rose thorns, cockleburrs, wood slivers, pieces of glass, tiny rocks, or other sharp objects imbedded in their footpads.

Also, they may be likely to catch one of their paws in a broken piece of wooden or chain-link fencing or even a small animal trap. Occasionally, a household pet may get his or her paw accidentally stepped-on if suddenly caught in the way of moving human feet. The extreme summer heat can also make asphalt very hot, which results in sore paws for some creatures.

How Rachel Treated Her Feline's Sore Paws

Rachel Emory was a third-year chemistry major at Vanderbilt University in Nashville when I met her some years ago. She related an intriguing tale of how her cat was treated for bruised paws. But the funny part of the story was the manner in which this cat had become injured.

It seems that her cat always had a habit of napping on a braided throw rug located directly behind a large rocking chair. One time a visitor accidentally sat down and commenced rocking before Rachel had time to warn him not to do so and well before the animal had time to scoot away from danger. The rather large person leaned back once and one of the curved rocker legs came down on poor pussy's paws. The cat let out a dreadful howl of pain and then gave a menacing hiss in the direction of the individual responsible for her suffering.

Rachel gathered up the injured cat in her arms, went into the kitchen and placed the animal on the kitchen table. She opened a cupboard and retrieved some arnica cream. With this she gently applied a small amount on each paw and very lightly rubbed it around. She then wrapped both paws in some loose gauze and held it in place with some adhesive tape. She repeated this process for the next several days. Within a week the bruises were gone and pussy was trotting around again as if nothing had happened. But after that, she completely avoided the rocking chair and never slept near it again.

What One Boy Did for His Dog's Sore Doggies

A boy I knew years ago by the name of Terry had a black Labrador puppy. One hot summer day he went skateboarding down a lone country road with his young dog in tow on a long lease behind him. The temperature was probably in the high nineties, but Terry wore sneakers and had no problem with the surface heat.

Unfortunately, his dog didn't have the same protection. After skate-boarding for a couple of hours, Terry went back home and noticed his dog limping behind him. He tried to get the animal to run in order to keep up with him. Finally, out of exasperation he had to carry both dog and skateboard the rest of the way.

He informed his mother of this and she told him that the poor puppy probably had burned his paws on the hot asphalt. So, the kid, on his own, went to the refrigerator and opened the top freezer door. He removed a tray of ice cubes and turned them into an empty plastic bowl. He took these and his dog outside with him and sat down on the back porch. He laid the pup in his lap and proceeded to dutifully rub each paw with an ice cube for a few minutes until the ice had pretty well melted. He then repeated the action again and again until all four paws had been thusly treated.

He set the dog down on the ground and watched with satisfaction as the pub walked around without any noticeable limping. Terry squatted down on his haunches, and the animal came over and licked one hand out of gratitude for what had been done to relieve its pain.

What's Good for Ferrets Is Good for Cats and Dogs

A friend of mine raises ferrets for a living. He told me of a simple remedy he sometimes had to apply if a few of them accidentally injured their footpads. He would rub some calendula cream on their paws, and within a couple of days the bruising would cease.

I've recommended this to different dog and cat owners with apparently good success. It's quick, easy, and inexpensive, but works quite well to heal injured paws. (See the Product Appendix under Nature's Answer to obtain any of these items.)

BUMPS & BRUISES

"Mother Nature's Ben Gay"

Dr. Bob Goldstein and his wife Susan have won the affection of many hundreds of dogs and cats in the Goldsteins' combined 40 years of animal care. He owns and operates a Connecticut veterinary clinic and she counsels in pet nutrition.

In the February 1997 issue of their newsletter, Susan wrote as follows: "Last winter, Annie (our Corgi) and I took a spill on a patch of ice. We nursed our aches, bumps and bruises. But we didn't reach for the Ben Gay (despite the fact that my mother and grandmother were practically addicted to the stuff). Instead, Bob rubbed us with what I call 'Mother Nature's Ben Gay,' Arnica gel.

"Once you try Arnica gel on yourself or your animals, you'll become a believer. For one thing, it's much cheaper and healthier than a shot of cortisone for stiffness and swelling. When your dog or cat falls or twists a limb, the body calls on its own rescue system. It sends blood into the injured area, which pushes against the walls of the capillaries releasing fluid into the area. This causes redness, swelling and painful pressure on the nerve endings. This topical homeopathic remedy focuses on treating the cause of the pain (swelling and inflammation), not suppressing the pain as many drugs do.

"Arnica gel contains Arnica montana, a plant that is used for an oral homeopathic remedy that speeds healing of bruises and relieves aches and pains. . . . Gels are so practical to use. They're easier to administer than a pill or capsule, and certainly in keeping with our resolution . . . to offer simple, healthful ways for you to care for the animals in your house.

"My favorite brand, ArniFlora from Boericke and Tafel, is also one of the most commonly available Arnica gels. You can buy it at health food stores and even some pharmacies.

"You may apply the gel up to four times daily (externally only) for bumps, bruises or joints that are stiff from over-exertion or arthritis. Part the hair and gently rub the gel directly on the skin. Avoid getting it into the eyes, and do not use ArniFlora if there is any break in the skin. If pain or swelling appear to worsen or persist for more than two or three days, see your veterinarian.

"I encourage you to keep a tube of Arnica gel in your home pharmacy and feel free to pair it up with the Arnica pellets that are taken internally for double the healing help."

Another Alternative: Mullein/ACV Fomentation

In various places throughout this text, I've stated my opposition to homeopathy. Out of respect for my friends Bob and Susan, though, I would encourage readers to use Arnica gel for its ease and simplicity. However, I feel obligated to offer a nonhomeopathic alter-

native that I've used for many years and with which I feel comfortable (since it squares with my philosophical beliefs).

One of the most common herbs found throughout much of the
U.S. and the lower part of Canada is mullein. This tall biennial plant
prefers waste places to grow in, that is, clearings, empty fields,
unused pastures, and alongside old highways and railroad tracks. Its
light-green leaves have an unmistakable velvetness to them.

Boil one pint consisting of equal parts (one cup each) of spring
water and apple-cider vinegar. Add two tablespoons of the finely cut
leaves. Cover and set aside to steep for 15 minutes. Strain the solution into another container. Make sure the solution is still quite hot.
Take an old but clean washcloth and dip it in, wringing out excess
liquid. Fold it over several times into a neat little pack and place
directly over the bump or bruise. On top of this apply a dry flannel
cloth and hold in place for several minutes until the cloth becomes
cool. Then repeat the process several times.

It is important to keep the animal still while doing this, preferably lying on its side. You'll be amazed at how quickly this remedy
works, but it is admittedly more cumbersome to do than Susan's suggestion. It takes more time, effort, and patience, while the other is
completed in a snap of the fingers. But this works along the line of
true herbal medicine and isn't homeopathic.

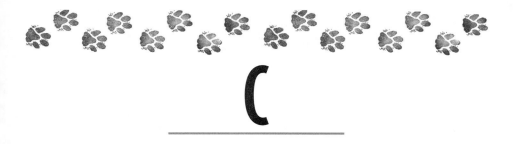

C

CANCER

Cancer Amid Biological Rationality

The simplest definition that can be given cancer, I suppose, is this: It is a disease event in which normal cells stop functioning and maturing properly. An accident occurs within them that is partly a change in their DNA or genetic blueprint. This is believed by some experts to be due to a type of biological "short" in electrical flow through the body. An unknown number of these extremely brief interruptions in electrical flow to healthy calls can wreak havoc with their DNA. The altered DNA makes copies of itself and passes its information and gene sequencing onto other cells, which then become cancer prone. As the normal cycle of cell creation and death experiences interference, the newly mutated cancer cells begin multiplying uncontrollably, no longer operating as an integrated and harmonious part of the body.

Think of the disease process another way. The human or animal body may be compared to a working computer. When everything is in good order, the machine runs smoothly. But if there is any kind of electrical disturbance within its framework, then it is usually said that "the computer is temporarily *down*." Nothing can be brought up on the screen when the keyboard is struck until the electrical glitch is corrected. And were it not for technological protection built within the computer itself, entire units of previously stored data might be forever lost. Sometimes, though, such safety devices don't always work as they should and a computer that "comes back on line" may occasionally continue to malfunction but without the full knowledge of its operator.

A similar pattern occurs at a cellular level. Healthy cells "talk" to one another through electrical impulses. When there is a "down" period, however brief, to this normal electrical flow, no communication happens between cells. If the delay is long enough or occurs too frequently, the DNA becomes scrambled for want of badly needed body electricity. This soon sets up a cell-mutation pattern that can eventually lead to cancer.

Basically speaking, cancer represents an accelerating process of inappropriate, uncontrolled cell growth. Think of it as "chaos amid biological rationality." When cancer cells are looked at in a high-powered electron microscope, they appear weird, to say the least. Their shapes are abnormal and their formations inconsistent. They are completely disorganized and contain misshapen internal structures, which is the essence of biological chaos.

In a nutshell, this is the most elementary explanation that could be given for the disease. These are the events leading up to and the results of cancers that occur in people and animals. While there will obviously be certain differences in human versus animal carcinomas, they both share a common pattern of electrical malfunction.

As Old as the Hills

Cancer in humans and domesticated animals is thought to be a modern epidemic. But the disease is actually quite old: Evidence of its presence has been detected in the mummified remains of nobility and some of their pets from Egypt and Peru that were embalmed nearly 5,000 years ago. The best reference for the Egyptian finds comes from the classic work edited by James E. Harris and Edward F. Wente, *An X-Ray Atlas of the Royal Mummies* (Chicago: University of Chicago Press, 1980). Pathological examination of some mummies of the ruling class showed definite tumors.

Other books on the subject have made brief references to "unusual growths" in mummified cats. The ancient Egyptians cherished animals and even mummified those deemed sacred. In their complex belief system, the cat portrayed Bastet, goddess of happiness. The pet *miu* (the Egyptian equivalent of house cat) led a life blessed by Bastet. And when a miu died, its owners shaved eyebrows in mourning and had their pet embalmed, wrapped in bandages, and laid to rest with deceased family members in their tombs. This is how we know that a few of these ancient felines probably had some type of cancer.

Wild dogs of the Old World called jackals also played a key role in Egyptian religion. When the renowned archaeologist Howard Carter was digging with his Egyptian workmen in the Valley of the Kings in November 1922, he uncovered a staircase. As the men cleared it, a doorway came into view affixed with royal seals bearing the jackal symbol of the god Anubis above nine defeated captives. "It was a thrilling moment for me," Carter later wrote. "Literally anything might lie beyond that passage, and it needed all my self-control to keep from breaking down the doorway, and investigating then and there."

But for nearly three agonizing weeks he waited for the arrival of a wealthy English nobleman, the Fifth Earl of Carnarvon (Lord Carnarvon) from London; he was the chap who was funding Carter's expedition. Then the clearing resumed. Finally, on November 26, 1922, they entered the tomb, where the glitter of gold and the sight of beautiful items made the onlookers strangely silent and subdued. Carter's reward was nothing short of spectacular. He had discovered the ancient tomb of Tutankhamun, the boy pharaoh who ruled Egypt for only a short time. "King Tut" became a household phrase overnight as the world press carried constant bulletins from the Valley of the Kings as the arduous labor continued. Today the wealth of Tutankhamun's tomb fills gallery after gallery in Cairo's Egyptian Museum.

But lesser known items of scientific value were carted from the tomb. Among them were the mummified remains of several small dogs, probably jackals. In the Egyptian faith of those times, Anubis was considered the god of embalming and assisting the dead to get into eternity. He was always drawn with a man's body, but a jackal's head. This was because, like the wild dogs who roamed graveyards at night, he communed with the dead. One of the two dogs taken from Tut's burial site was pathologically examined many years later and found to have had an unexplained growth of "substantial size" on the left side of its abdomen.

Although the evidence is somewhat meager, it does seem to indicate that at least in a few instances, cats and dogs may have suffered from incidental tumors several millennia ago in the Land of the Nile. But the occurrence of cancer then was nowhere near the explosive proportions it is now in current veterinary practice. This is undoubtedly due to the fact that household pets then ate table scraps free from chemical contaminants.

Cell Normalization with an Ancient Herb?

Several medical and pharmaceutical writings from ancient China seem to suggest that cancer was prevalent there as well, but not in the runaway proportions seen now in people and pets. Two of the best treatises on the subject of disease and healing are *Sheng Nung Ben Cao Chien* or *The Herbal Classic of the Divine Plowman* and *Huang Ti Nei Chien*. While the authors are unknown, both works were written around 100 B.C. The *Herbal Classic* contains three volumes describing 365 drugs—one for each day of the year. Among them, 252 are derived from plants, 67 from animals, and 46 from minerals. The book describes the properties of each drug in detail, including its taste, source of collection, pharmacological action, and therapeutic uses.

This book also outlines approximately 170 types of diseases that are effectively treated with these 365 herbs. Some of the descriptions have been proven to be correct and accurate by recent scientific investigations. For example, ginseng was said to "strengthen mentality, relax stress, and calm the nerves . . ." It is now known that the active principles of ginseng, panaxosides, do exert effects on the central nervous system and the cardiovascular system and stimulate the adeno-corticotropic hormone-cortisol axis.

Furthermore, the *Herbal Classic* mentioned the root being good for "increasing body fortification against wasting sickness and reducing growths of exceptional size." Scientists who've worked with the root in laboratories and used extracts of it on animal models now know that small doses of ginseng saponins from either the root or leaf can reduce tumor weight. Ginseng is capable of stimulating the production of specific antibodies in animals, resulting in an increase of immune function. Ginsenosides were found to be particularly effective in the treatment of cancer patients, improving their appetites and aiding in sleep. Objective signs such as a decrease in tumor size and increase of serum immunoglobulins have also been observed in those patients treated with ginseng.

For our purposes here, though, it may be worthwhile mentioning that *before* the herb was used on human subjects it was first tested on animal models. Mongrel dogs with chemically induced tumors were fed extracts of ginseng-root powder in their daily rations. A 45-percent reduction in tumors was observed. Interestingly, ginseng *tea* given to cats with cancer in place of water worked better in reducing tumors than did the powdered root extract.

The active ginsenosides are decidedly antioxidant. Other experimental data have shown that giving ginsenosides to animals inoculated with S-180 cancer cells can prolong animal survival. The mechanism of the anticancer activity of ginsenosides isn't well understood, however. When ginsenosides were added to the culture medium of cancer cells, a morphological change of the cancer cells was noticed. The number of cytosol mitochondria increased significantly and they were arranged in a more orderly fashion. It appears that the ginsenosides can to some extent reduce the biological chaos in cells when there are momentary disruptions in their electrical supply. At a concentration of 2.5 to 5 milligrams per milliliter, ginseng alcoholic extract can inhibit the growth of S-180 or U-14 cancer cells in the culture media.

The *Yellow Emperor's Classic of Internal Medicine* (the other Chinese treatise cited earlier) teaches that *chi* is the life energy that permeates the entire universe, this planet, and every living thing therein. There are cycles to everything, a constant rhythmic shifting, if you will, from one pole to its opposite. And just as every process of nature shows cyclicity, every process has a polar nature. Though oneness is the primary law of the universe, this fundamental two-dimensional view of nature generates the concept of *yin* and *yang*. This great principle provides a basis for comprehending the fundamental pattern of all processes.

Cycles occur as phenomena oscillate rhythmically between energetically actives phases and resting states. The *Huang Ti Nei*

Chien explains that when all phenomena is in the overtly active stage of its cycle, then it is said to be in a yang mode. Conversely, all phenomena in its covert, quietistic stage are reckoned to be yin. Put another way: Yin conserves while yang radiates.

The process of cancer in animals or humans is a relatively simple one when examined by this kind of philosophical logic. When there is an obstruction in the steady flow of chi, it invariably produces an imbalance between the yin and yang states. This leads to reduced blood circulations and less effective elimination of waste materials. All these factors, it is believed, lead to the development of cancer.

What ginseng root can do, by this rationale, is to remove chi obstructions and thereby help to restore balance between the yin and yang in higher life forms. It also enhances circulations and increases bowel and bladder activity, which remove accumulated toxins from the system.

Ginseng can be administered to a sick animal one of several different ways. A non-alcoholic fluid extract of ten drops may be squirted into the animal's mouth by holding the jaws apart with a gloved hand and using the other one to accomplish this. When giving to cats, though, remember to cut a hole in an old, heavy bath towel and to drape it over the feline first to prevent claw scratching.

Capsules are of proven worth in cancer treatment, too. I find that a blend of Korean ginseng root with Japanese aged garlic extract gets better results many times than if plain ginseng were used. Empty the contents of two gelatin capsules (for a small ten-pound animal) or double this amount (for a larger sized one) into the food of an ailing pet and mix thoroughly before serving. Do this twice daily. (See the Product Appendix under Wakunaga of America for more information.)

Ginseng tea is another matter. Some animals will take to it, but others won't. Dogs seem to dislike the tea more than cats do. I've found that if some catnip is added to the root tea, it should help persuade finicky felines to drink the mixture. Boil one pint of water and add one-and-a-half teaspoons of dried, cut ginseng root. Cover, lower the heat, and simmer for several minutes, then set aside. Uncover and add one-half teaspoon dried catnip herb, stir, replace the lid and permit to seep for 30 minutes. Strain half of this and refrigerate the rest for a later serving.

EMFs: Another Potential Health Threat for Pets and People

In preparation of this book, I learned something I wasn't expecting: how very little pet care authorities know on some matters while having extensive knowledge in other areas. This became apparent as I scanned the available pet-care books and magazines for material on EMFs, or electromagnetic fields. Virtually *nothing* could be found on the subject in any of the current best-sellers or major magazines such as *Cat Fancy, Dog Fancy,* or *Natural Pet.* Yes, some of them did talk about polluted air, chlorinated/fluoridated tap water, and chemically contaminated soft-moist and other pet foods as leading factors in the cause of small animal cancers. But not one addressed the real threat of EMFs.

EMFs are invisible lines of force that surround all electrical devices and wiring. Concern about their possible negative health impact was catalyzed in the late 1970s by many studies linking childhood leukemia and proximity to certain types of power lines or equipment, such as utility transformers. (Might there not be a probable connection of some kind between feline leukemia and cats who rest near home computers or color televisions that are on and running?)

More recently, other sources have been added: large currents on the job, poorly grounded wiring, and numerous household and office appliances. EMFs don't necessarily correlate with the size, power, or noisiness of a device. Moreover, there can be a tremendous difference between models of an appliance. Because it is exceedingly hard to shield oneself or a pet from EMFs, the only practical way to limit exposures is to put distance between oneself and the pet with that of the source.

A somewhat pricy device known as a gaussmeter is available to consumers to measure the electromagnetic fields present in their homes or offices. The following table was compiled from data supplied to this author by the National Institute of Environmental Health Sciences and the Department of Energy. It gives you a good idea of EMFs generated by a variety of electrical devices and machines.

EMFs FOR ORDINARY ELECTRICAL APPLIANCES
(MEASURED IN MILLIGAUS UNITS)

Electrical Appliances	Actual Distance from Pet/Pet Owner	
	(six inches)	(one foot)
HAIR DRYER		
highest	700	70
lowest	1	undetectable
DISHWASHER		
highest	100	30
lowest	10	7
IRON		
highest	23	2
lowest	5	1
VACUUM CLEANER		
highest	710	204
lowest	97	19
PHOTOCOPIER		
highest	207	38
lowest	3	1
COLOR TELEVISION		
highest	22	9
lowest	undetectable	undetectable
AIR CONDITIONER (window)		
highest	18	7
lowest	2	undetectable
COMPUTER SCREEN		
highest	24	8
lowest	9	4

In late November 1997, a U.S. Public Health Service conference was held in Washington, D.C. It was devoted exclusively to the biological influences that EMFS could exert on humans and household animals. A number of studies presented by different scientists gave new evidence showing that the cells and tissues of pets and people are extremely responsive to such invisible magnetic fields.

One of the more interesting facts brought out was that such fields exert effects upon and through hormones. Take the widely known brain hormone melatonin. It is an important natural suppressor of cancer-cell growth, both in test tubes and in various animals. EMFs can severely depress or even close down melatonin reduction in small animals. This can then help to foster tumor growths.

Toxicologist Wolfgang Löscher of the School of Veterinary Medicine in Hanover, Germany, reported exposing a group of 120 female rats to melatonin-suppressing EMFs of between 100 and 1,000 mG (milliGaus). An equal number of rats received a negligible background exposure of roughly 1 mG; these rats produced melatonin normally. Löscher then injected into each rodent a chemical that induces mammary cancer and kept the rats under observation for three months.

Compared with the unexposed rats, those in the 100-mG field developed about 10 percent more tumors. Animal models exposed to 500 mG got 25 percent more cancer. And rats getting zapped with 1,000 mG developed 50 percent more cancer. Malignancies also grew as much as twice the size under the influence of these electromagnetic fields.

Herbal Protection Against EMFs

There is one principal category of herbs that definitely afford protection to pets and people against electromagnetic-field radiation. These are cultivated grasses, more notably cereal grasses such as wheat and barley grasses and red-clover blossoms. Some years ago I started using both on a regular basis for staying healthy. At the time I had my office cat named Jake, I also gave him adequate amounts of these grasses in powdered form.

Now, one may be inclined to ask, "What evidence did you have that it protected your pet from potential cancer such as feline leukemia?" My response would be, "From one of observation." This particular cat, you see, had a frequent habit of resting on the top covers of our two office photocopy machines, especially while they were turned on. Perhaps it was the electrical warmth or the low-intensity sounds they generated or maybe a combination of both that attracted him to them. For whatever unknown reason, Jake really liked those machines a lot. After a while it got to be a regular joke with all who came into our research center. The first inquiry would usually be something like, "Say, where's that copy cat of yours?" One of my secretaries even bought a small oval-shaped fabric cover that she placed on top of the larger copier lid. Jake found this most comfortable and spent more time relaxing on this machine.

Many times in the evening while I worked at my desk he would come over and lie just a few inches away from my word processor. Sometimes, in bolder moments, he would even have the audacity to walk *across* the keyboard while I had a sheet of paper still in it and type his own gibberish. He clearly was master of his own domain, and I often yielded to him on this point.

I would venture to say that over a period of several years while having the constant run of our research center, this animal was zapped with enough EMF radiation to last several cats many lifetimes. And yet, never once did he show any signs of leukemia or other malignancies as one would expect under such unusual circumstances.

As I look back on the matter, I'm convinced that adding one-quarter teaspoon of wheat-grass powder and the contents of two capsules of red-clover blossoms every day to his moist food was what saved him from getting sick. (See the Product Appendix under Pines International for cereal grasses.) These food supplements surely afforded him protection against such invisible lines of deadly force. Without doubt his cells were being bombarded on a regular basis with high amounts of electromagnetic waves. And yet not one of Jake's proverbial nine lives was ever phased with cancer. This, to me, surely was the greatest testimony of all with regard to the outstanding nutritional contents of such field grasses that shielded my cat from potentially damaging electrical radiation.

And while I've worked a lot with wheat grass juice and red clover tea in humans with cancer who've sought my free advice in such matters, *never once* have I known a dog or cat similarly afflicted with the same disease ever to take to these items in liquid form. It is only in the powders intermingled with their regular food that they've willingly consumed such things without making a fuss.

Other Causes of Cancer in Pets

In *Dr. Pitcairn's Complete Guide to Natural Health for Dogs & Cats* (Emmaus, PA: Rodale Press, Inc., 1995), the author, a renowned veterinarian, lists a number of other factors that could expose a family dog or cat to possible carcinogens. "These include," he writes, "cigarette smoke, riding in the back of a pickup truck (and inhaling car fumes) . . . drinking water from street puddles (which can contain hydrocarbons and asbestos dust from brakes), frequent diagnostic work with x-rays (all radiation effects are cumulative in the body), use of strong toxic chemicals over long periods (as with flea and tick control) and consuming pet foods high in organ meats and meat meal (concentrators of pesticides, and growth hormones used to fatten cattle, which can promote cancer growth) as well as in preservatives and artificial colors known to cause cancer in lab animals."

He insists that "a fresh natural diet is imperative" to cancer prevention in pets. He recommends that it be supplemented "with vitamins C, A and E as well as yeast and fresh raw vegetables (particularly sprouts and grasses, notable for their B vitamin and trace mineral contents)." Use a little imagination and fix your cat or dog vegetable meat loaf, which could include salmon or sardines (for the feline) or lamb or young beef (for the canine). One teaspoon of Rex's Wheat Germ Oil in such a vegetable meat loaf or mixed in with other food every day will provide all the vitamin E needed. (See the Product Appendix under Anthropological Research Center to order this particular item.) Different types of sprouts may be made at home with the help of books on the subject. (My *Heinerman's Encyclopedia of Nuts, Berries, and Seeds,* from the same publisher as this book, provides detailed information on sprouting.) And cereal grasses, of course, may be obtained in bulk powder to add to a pet's regular food. (See the Product Appendix under Pines.)

A Tucson, Arizona, company has gone to great research expense to formulate what I consider to be some top-of-the-line dry packaged and moist canned foods for your cat or dog. Meat sources include organically raised lamb, beef, and chicken, ocean fish, and unconventional but healthful poultry such as ostrich and emu. These are balanced with plant proteins obtained from barley, oatmeal, alfalfa, flax seed, and mesquite bean. A variety of essential vitamins, minerals, amino acids, and herbs have also been added to these products. In my diligent hunt throughout North America for prepared pet foods that I could recommend *in good conscience,* I came across these while attending the Natural Products Expo East convention in Baltimore in September 1997. One of the owners, Lisa Newman, told me, "We wanted pet foods good enough for even the owners to eat if they had to!" Now that's a bold statement to make to underscore the remarkable quality of these products. (See the Product Appendix under Holistic Animal Care for more information.)

Dr. Pitcairn offers several wise suggestions for owners to follow while their pets are receiving conventional cancer therapy (a position I'm not at all in favor of).

- Totally avoid commercial foods. "Feed only fresh, unprocessed foods."

- Administer large amounts of vitamin C every day. He recommends giving 1,000 mg. "for every 15 pounds of body weight" and dividing it in half between the morning and evening.

- *Never* use tap water!

- Do not submit your animal for *any* type of immunizations. Be stubborn and flatly refuse your vet's suggestions in this thing. "Giving a vaccine to an animal with cancer," Dr. Pitcairn writes, is the equivalent of "pouring gasoline on a fire."

After all is said and done, cancer in animals is generally met with greater patience and far less anxiety than in people. Animals have an incredible tolerance for pain and suffering that exceeds even what the strongest and stoutest of humans could put up with. This is something that has amazed me through the years. And, to this day, I'm still in awe at how wonderfully well a cat or dog can meet this disease and do it with such class and dignity. We who are supposed to be the higher evolved species can take some lessons from the fine examples that noble souls within the animal kingdom have set for us as a worthy course to follow when we may become sick sometime in our own lives.

The World's Two Best Anticancer Herbal Formulas

"Every year medical science spends billions of dollars in a desperate search for the cure—or cures—for cancer. And yet, despite the use of increasingly expensive and dangerous technology and drugs, we never seem to get any closer to sparing mankind from our most dreaded and deadly disease.

"Is it possible that the answer to our prayers about treating cancer has been available to us all along, a gift from nature, hidden in the life-giving properties of certain plants that grow wild all over North America?

"The answer is yes."

So begins the advertising blurb on the front inside flap of the dust-jacket cover for the book *Calling of an Angel* (Los Angeles: Silent Walker Publishing, 1988) by Dr. Gary I. Glum. This is a biographical account of the late Rene Caisse, RN (who lived to the ripe old age of 90) the discoverer of an old Native American herbal cancer cure that she eventually dubbed "Essiac" (her name spelled backwards).

For over half a century, this woman "successfully treated thousands of cancer patients" with an herbal concoction that Canadian Indians had been using for many centuries for the same disease. In 1983–1984, doctors at the University of Toronto's Hospital for Sick Children began testing Essiac on eight of ten patients with surgically treated tumors of the central nervous system that had "escaped from the conventional methods of therapy including both radiation and chemotherapy."

Dr. E. Bruce Hendrick, the head neurosurgeon who initiated this program, stated his reasons for doing so in a letter to the Canadian Minister of Health and Welfare. "I am most impressed with the effectiveness of the treatment and its lack of side effects. . . . I feel that this method of treatment should be given serious consideration and would benefit from a scientific clinical trial."

The other popular and equally successful cancer treatment using nothing but natural substances is the Hoxsey Therapy. Richard Walters writes in the opening paragraph of his ninth chapter in *Options: The Alternative Cancer Therapy Book* (New York: Avery Publishing Group, Inc., 1993): "For over three decades, Harry Hoxsey (1901–1974), a self-taught healer, cured many cancer patients using an herbal remedy reported handed down by his great-grandfather. By the 1950s, the Hoxsey Cancer Clinic in Dallas was the world's largest private cancer center, with branches in seventeen states. Born in Illinois, the charismatic practitioner of herbal folk medicine faced unrelenting opposition and harassment from a hostile medical establishment. Nevertheless, two federal courts upheld the 'therapeutic value' of Hoxsey's internal tonic. Even his archenemies, the American Medical Association and the Food and Drug Administration, admitted that his treatment could cure some forms of cancer. A Dallas judge ruled in federal court that Hoxsey's therapy was 'comparable to surgery, radium, and x-ray' in its effectiveness, without the destructive side effects of those treatments.' But in the 1950s, at the tail end of the McCarthy era, Hoxsey's clinics were shut down. The AMA, NCI [National Cancer Institute], and FDA organized a 'conspiracy' to 'suppress' a fair, unbiased assessment of Hoxsey's methods, according to a 1953 federal report to Congress."

In my own scientific research with alternative-medicine options spanning several decades, I have become familiar with both Essiac and the Hoxsey Formula. I devote a number of pages to both of them years ago in *The Treatment of Cancer with Herbs* (Orem, UT: BiWorld Publishers, 1980). In that book I attempt to show that they were good not only for human cancers but also for those afflicting animals as well. Since that time, I have recommended one or the other or both to hundreds of pet owners worldwide who've had animals suffering from a variety of tumors. Individually and sometimes used together, both have had a high rate of success in sending this disease into partial or total remission.

Nurse Caisse's formula is relatively simple: burdock root, sheep sorrel, slippery-elm bark, and turkey rhubarb root. Equal parts (three-quarters cup) of burdock, sorrel, and rhubarb is simmered in one gallon of distilled or purified water for ten minutes. After this, it is set aside, uncovered, and one cup of slippery elm added. The contents are vigorously stirred, the lid put back on, and everything is permitted to steep for one hour. Essentially, that's how Rene made her tea: She used only dried, coarsely cut botanicals and never any powdered materials. These items are available from most health-food stores or herbal companies such as Indiana Botanic Gardens in Hammond, Indiana, and don't cost very much.

Harry's formula, on the other hand, has always been a bit more complex, somewhat in keeping with the man's own quirky personality. As cited in my own book years ago, "the AMA had a laboratory analysis done of a 16 ox. bottle of the liquid Hoxsey 'Cancer' Tonic. Each 5 cc. was found to contain the following ingredients: potassium iodine 150 mg., licorice 20 mg., red clover, 20 mg., burdock root, 10 mg., stillingia root, 10 mg., berberis root (barberry), 10 mg., poke root, 10 mg., cascara sagrada, 5 mg., prickly ash bark, 5 mg., and buckthorn bark, 20 mg. A tea similar to the one Nurse Caisse used has been made from the ingredients, as well as an alcohol fluid extract."

A Hungarian pharmacist in Calgary, Canada, has taken much of the guesswork, fuss, and time out of each formula preparation by manufacturing it in ready-to-use liquid supplements. Gavriel Harel and his father before him (who was also a pharmacist) have been in business since 1921 making liquid herbal extracts for animal and human use. (See the Product Appendix under Flora Beverage Co., Ltd. for more on Essex Botanical and Hoxsiac Herbal Drink.)

The amount to be given an animal depends, of course, on its size. For cats, either tea or the manufactured liquid supplement should be given in twice-daily, 10-drop allotments. Cut a hole in an old bath towel and fit it over the cat's head; this will protect you against being scratched. Wearing a leather glove on one hand, gently force open the feline's mouth and squirt the liquid toward the back. Do this in the morning and again in the evening until the disease shows evidence of remission. The same dosage applies for small dogs. For large canines, double this amount and administer twice daily.

What Sharks Know that We Don't Know

Before the dinosaurs roamed the earth, paleontologists tell us, sharks swam in the ancient seas. Long after *T. rex,* sharks were still in existence. Then came the big woolly mammoths and saber-toothed tigers. What the Ice Age didn't claim, the La Brea tar pits in Los Angeles (and similar deposits elsewhere) eventually got. But the sharks continued undisturbed in the defiant role as ocean predators. In the meantime, different species of men evolved, acquiring more skills with their advancing intelligences. But even some of them took "wrong turns" on the human highway and wound up in what eventually proved to be the genetic equivalent of dead-end streets. We need only recall what happened to the suddenly extinct Neanderthal race to know the reality of this. However, sharks thrived and let nothing interfere with their existence. Today there we are here along with everything that is contemporary to the animal kingdom. But in light of our recent nuclear capabilities and awesome potential for self-destruction some-day, we, too, might become just a blip on the screen of life . . . but the sharks will probably *still* manage somehow to swim on!

It can be correctly said of any shark that has ever lived that that creature doesn't have a single bone in its body. Most animals, including ourselves, have skeletons composed of calcified bone. The skeletons of sharks, however, are composed of pure cartilage, a hard gristly material formed from proteins and complex carbohydrates and toughened by rodlike fibers. And did you know that between 6 and 8 percent of a shark's gross weight is cartilage, while just a tiny fraction of 1 percent of a mammal's gross weight is cartilage?

In 1976 a scientist named Dr. Robert Langer began investigating isolated factors of shark cartilage to see whether or not it had any antitumor potential. His report was published in the journal *Science* (193:70-72) for that year. In 1981 CNN (Cable News Network) became the first media source to break the story of his remarkable discovery. I remember watching cable TV that day and seeing this bold announcement flash upon the screen every 30 minutes: "Shark cartilage cures cancer." In 1992 another researcher, Dr. I. William Lane, wrote the book *Sharks Don't Get Cancer* (Garden City Park, NY: Avery Publishing Group, Inc.), which became an overnight best-seller and set the medical, pharmaceutical, and health-food-supplement industries on their ears. Probably no single substance in recent memory has made such a tremendous impact on the health psyches of consumers worldwide as this has.

Right after shark cartilage, the research on shark liver oil began pouring in from scientists everywhere. A unique group of compounds collectively called alkylglycerols were tested in dogs and other small animals and shown to have remarkable anticancer properties, too, but in ways somewhat different from that for shark cartilage.

Pet owners intending to use either shark-derived substance for the benefit of animals stricken with cancer should look around for the best quality available. Shark cartilage and shark liver oil work better together than they do alone. (See the Product Appendix under Scandinavian Naturals for shark supplements.)

CONJUNCTIVITIS

A Remedy from Scotland

Some years ago a friend of mine, Robert Dunbar of Scotland, sent me the following clipping as it appeared in the *Glasgow Herald,* a newspaper of some antiquity and considerable influence. Unfortunately, he didn't write down the day, month, year, or page. But his letter, bearing a March 6, 1979, postmark may suggest a likely date within the first quarter of that year, perhaps.

Cleaning Purulent Matter from Small-Animal Eyes

Glasgow—To hear Theron Dunkirk, a small-animal practitioner tell it, all you need are a few medicinal plants to concoct a simple eye remedy. In a public lecture held last night in Yardley Hall, the good doctor devoted considerable time to proclaiming the virtues of plants over conventional agents in treating small animals.

The attentive crowd of some 175 listened eagerly as he told them how to make an eye wash for animals with conjunctivitis. His favorites for this are mint leaves, fennel seed, and spikes of brilliantly colored gladiola flowers. His method of preparation begs description.

"Pour a small teapot of boiling water over a tablespoonful of fennel seeds," he said. These he would cover with a lid to "let simmer a few minutes." The mint and gladiolas were added afterwards and covered again. After steeping for awhile, the contents were to be strained into another vessel.

"The eyes of any afflicted animal can then be rinsed out with this solution," he noted. Cotton was the best material to use for doing so. "It should always be used while lukewarm," he reminded everyone. This way the gluey matter could be more easily removed from the eyes and eyelids.

Some of the audience wished to know if this could also be applicable to similar conditions in young children.

"I can't see where this would hurt any," Mr. Dunkirk observed. "I've been using it on my own little ones and haven't seen evidence of any harmful effects on their eyes. . . ."

His presentation was compelling and stirred in the memories of many, reflections on those times when their own parents and grandparents used such nostrums for their own needs, as well as those of their own animals in some certain cases.

(For additional information from the same article, see the entry under Red Eye.)

CONSTIPATION

Stress- or Diet-Induced

Constipation is frequent among animals that are subjected to a lot of tension or that receive insufficient bulk fiber in their diets. Also, inadequate exercise may lead to blocked or sluggish bowels. If a pet isn't permitted to evacuate when the urge is present, it could develop the unfortunate habit of holding its stool.

Put another way, some of the same factors that lead to constipation in people do the same with pets. Animal bodies respond similarly to stress and poor diets, in much the same way our systems do. And the solutions are about the same, too.

Natural Laxatives

Olive oil is safe and tonifying for animal colons. Not only will it stimulate intestinal muscle contractions, but it also tends to lubricate impacted fecal mass. Mix one-half (cats) to one (dog) teaspoon of extra-virgin olive oil twice a day in both feedings until regular movements become evident again.

Mixing one-half to one teaspoon of powdered psyllium seed (depending on the animal's size) in the food twice daily promotes bowel activity in a hurry. You can get this herb in health-food stores. It is completely safe and not habit-forming.

Feeding animals fresh or dried fruits that are naturally sweet tasting always guarantees colon activity within hours. Figs, dates, prunes, bananas, and even berries work wonders.

Wheat or barley grass make ideal laxatives, too. Mix one-half teaspoon (cats) to one tablespoon (dogs) in with every feeding. (See Product Appendix under Pines International for additional information.)

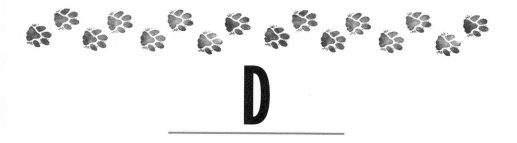

D

Diabetes

Near Epidemic Proportions

In a number of previous health encyclopedias geared for people, I've always included discussions on diabetes and ways to cope with it. For some time I've said that this has been an insidiously quiet disease on the verge of becoming a national epidemic. The statistics speak for themselves

- Sixteen million Americans have diabetes.
- Ninety-three percent of these cases are over 40 and have Type II.
- Thirteen percent of Americans between the ages of 65 and 74 have diabetes.
- Diabetes is the nation's fourth leading cause of death. It kills an estimated 300,000 people every year in the United States alone.
- Diabetes is the leading cause of foot amputations, accounting for about half of all such amputations (60,000 annually) other than those performed as a result of accidents.
- Every year, 15 percent of U.S. health-care dollars—$100 billion— is spent on the treatment of this disease.

When I commenced research for this natural pet care book a couple of years ago, I quickly learned to my astonishment that this same problem ranks as one of the leading diseases in small animals. Practically every veterinarian I interviewed by phone or in person from coast to coast put diabetes at or near the top of their lists for what they regularly see in many of their patients. "It's a biggee!" one Atlanta-based veterinary practitioner told me. And a West Coast veterinarian summed it up another way: "Diabetes is right up there among the top five most common disorders that come through our clinic doors every day."

The Sugar Fix

When I asked Dr. JoAnne Stefanatos, owner and operator of the Animal Kingdom Veterinary Hospital in Las Vegas, Nevada, for her professional opinion on why this disease is growing at an alarming rate in dogs and cats, she was forthright and definite in her remarks.

"Count birds in there, too," she began. When I interrupted her out of surprise for an explanation, she added: "So far I've seen several parakeets with diabetes. It's because their seed foods are sugary and filled with preservatives. What else would you expect?"

She sees the problem all the time in older canines and felines, "usually those eight years or older." She blames the commercial pet foods and owners' irresponsibility for most of it. "There is just too much sugar in everything. You can't buy a decent brand of [pet] food anymore without there being some kind of sugar in it. An animal's system will rebel just like the human body does when excess sugar is taken into it. The same autoimmune disorder that attacks human pancreatic cells that make insulin destroys the insulin-producing capabilities in our dogs and cats."

This "oversugarfying" of everything, as she puts it, goes beyond the supermarket to include owner indiscretions at feeding a favorite pet sugary treats for emotional or reward purposes. "That is about the worst thing that could be done," she emphasized. "It's like giving your baby sugar cubes to suck on. It introduces the pet to a substance that clearly creates a druglike dependency within the system. The animal finds it irresistible and will do just about anything to please its owner in order to get more of the same."

But "oversugarfying" and owner irresponsibility, while certainly major contributing factors to diabetes, do not form the entire picture. An equal amount of blame must be laid to the numerous chemical additives and preservatives included with most commercial pet foods these days. Dr. Stefanatos's view is shared by another holistic veterinarian, Dr. Tejinder Sodhi, who has been in practice for 15 years and operates the Animal Wellness Center in Bellevue, Washington.

Both animal-care professionals weren't at all reticent about vocalizing their strong opinions about this matter. Dr. Tejinder: "There are way too many chemicals in pet food that no one knows the side effects of. And the rancid fat that is used to cook a lot of this food that pets eat only complicates things more." Dr. Stefanatos: "The pesticides, preservatives, and additives in pet food *reprogram* the organs so their functions behave differently. No one knows the full extent of the problem, but it's there, nevertheless."

The Nature of Animal Diabetes

The most common form of this disease in small animals is uncomplicated diabetes mellitus, which is similar in many ways to that seen in humans. There are two types: Type I requires daily insulin, while Type II doesn't need it. Early signs include voluminous discharge of urine in a given period, chronic excessive intake of water, gluttony, and weight loss. Later symptoms include loss of appetite, laziness, depression, and vomiting. Obesity with recent weight loss is typical for most cases.

Sometimes canines may develop cataracts in later stages of the disease. Cats commonly experience dorsal muscle wasting and an oily coat with dandruff. Both species are also prone to liver enlargement, but jaundice is more prevalent in cats, as a rule. Cats occasionally develop diabetic neuropathy, but not that often.

The name of the disease is derived from a Greek word meaning *siphon* and the Latin word *mellitus,* meaning honey-sweet. It is aptly named because the passage of large amounts of sugar-laden urine is a key characteristic of poorly controlled diabetes.

Diabetes is a metabolic disorder: It results from an inability of the animal (or human) body to properly utilize glucose for energy needs. All of the carbohydrates and some protein components (amino acids) in foods are converted into glucose by an animal's body. Normally, glucose travels from the bloodstream into the cells under the influence of insulin, a hormone produced in the beta cells of the pancreas. Once inside the cell, glucose is immediately used as fuel for various metabolic functions. It is stored for later use as glycogen in the liver and muscles. Or, following conversion to triglycerides, it winds up in the fat tissue. Insulin also prevents the liver from forming glucose from amino acids and cuts the excessive breakdown of adipose-tissue triglycerides, which can put an animal into a human-type of diabetic coma.

In diabetes, insulin is either absent or its action is impaired. In either case, glucose can't enter the cells as it should. The result in both types of diabetes is that blood-sugar levels remain extremely high. After each meal, ingested carbohydrate elevates blood glucose; between meals, the liver makes excess glucose.

The Causes

Animal diabetes is believed by many veterinarians to be an autoimmune disorder just as in people. The animal body produces antibodies that attack and damage the pancreatic beta cells. At first, the ability of the beta cells to secrete insulin is merely impaired. Eventually, though, they stop secreting insulin altogether (this happens in a year or less). Fortunately, the tissues in pets with Type I respond normally to insulin delivered by injection and these animals must receive it daily from their owners.

Resistance to insulin is common in obesity and is a uniform feature of Type II. In this disorder, an animal's body tissues (primarily the muscles) become less sensitive to insulin action. In order to get cells the glucose they need, the beta cells of the pancreas must increase their production of insulin. Diabetes results when the beta cells are unable to secrete enough extra insulin to overcome the tissue resistance. Most animal cases with Type II can be treated with diet modification, herbs, nutrients, and other modalities. Only about 25 percent of them need insulin to achieve adequate control of their blood sugar.

Animals may develop this disease as a result of some other disorder. For example, diabetes can result from diseases that destroy pancreatic beta cells, such as chronic pancreatitis (more common in small, overweight, middle-aged dogs and Siamese cats). Endocrine cancer can, likewise, induce diabetes through the overproduction of hormones that interfere with insulin action. Much more common, though, is that certain drugs can induce diabetes or uncover it in borderline cases.

There is growing evidence that diabetes may also be triggered by a viral infection. The virus under suspicion seems to be an endogenous retrovirus, which is capable of infection in both animals and people. This retrovirus is usually dormant within the system, but can become activated through emotional, immunological, environmental, or dietary stresses. Once this happens a type of protein or protein fragment known as a superantigen goes into production. This, in turn, stimulates the activity of a large number of normally quiescent immune cells that then begin attacking the pancreas for no apparent reason. This rather novel research originated in Switzerland and was published in *Science News* (152:218), October 4, 1997.

Dietary Approaches

Diabetes in animals or people can in many instances be successfully managed with dietary modifications. For our purposes here, however, the discussion is confined to just animals, though some of the suggestions undoubtedly apply to humans.

Avoid giving diabetic animals soft, moist foods in plastic bags that don't need refrigeration. They tend to be high in sugar, artificial flavorings and colors, and chemical preservatives. Even healthy animals do poorly on this type of fare.

If the animal is obese, a gradual weight reduction is vital. This can be done in one of two ways. The first is to reduce the caloric intake to 60 percent (canines) or 70 percent (felines) of the caloric requirement for the animal's ideal body weight. The second method is to feed the pet a high-fiber, low-calorie food in a quantity similar to what the animal is accustomed. The weight loss should be achieved within a three-month period, if possible. Rapid weight loss is bad, especially in diabetic cats since they are prone to abnormal accumulations of fats within their liver cells (called hepatic lipidosis).

The role of fiber is critical to safe and successful weight loss and obesity prevention. Another beneficial effect is improved glycemic control. Fiber also promotes regularity, which does away with con-stipation in many obese animals. The best diet should always be high in fiber, low in fat, and high in complex carbohydrates.

Nonobese dogs and cats should be fed a consistent diet that they can be counted on to eat. It wouldn't be a bad idea for the owner to keep the daily caloric intake at a constant level and not vary it too much. Diabetic animals that have become thin as a result of their disease should receive *extra* calories. By denying them such, owners run the risk of creating an acidosis condition whereby alka-line reserves are depleted and immune functions severely impaired.

Animals that must receive twice-daily insulin injections or oral-ly administered hypoglycemic agents should be fed twice a day; each feeding should coincide with an insulin treatment. But for ani-mals on once-daily insulin, half the food may be given with the injection and the remainder in another eight hours. For nibblers, dry food can be randomly fed, and two small meals of wholesome moist food can given.

Both Drs. Stefanatos and Sodhi advocate diets that are high in fiber and consist of quality protein. Lightly steamed vegetables such as carrots, pea pods, broccoli, string beans, or cauliflower, baked tubers such as yams or potatoes (with the skin intact), canned pumpkin or squash, or certain salad greens provide the necessary roughage. Sources of good protein would be cooked or boiled eggs, cooked or canned salmon (no tuna fish here), and tofu.

Green bean and pea pods and Jerusalem artichoke hearts are particularly good for animal diabetes as they contain substances that are closely related to or mimic insulin.

Another wonderful source of fiber are the cereal grains: corn-meal, rye, barley, oats, rice, millet, quinoa, and wheat. They can be cooked, flavored with a few drops of pure vanilla, and served luke-warm or cold. Or the powders of some of these can be worked into other food and given in that manner. (See the Product Appendix under Pines for more information.)

Some veterinarians believe that dairy products are helpful since they are alkalizing and can overcome diabetic acidosis situations. I don't recommend giving an animal store-bought milk but only the fresh kind if it's available. If not then resort to goat's milk (fresh, canned, or packaged) or soy milk.

Nutritional Supplements

Dr. Sodhi utilizes a variety of different nutritional supplements on his animal patients. Some may be mixed with food, but others cannot. Some products work well for both cats and dogs, but others can be given only to felines. Dogs, he has discovered, "respond better to nutritional therapy than cats do." On the other hand, "diet modification works better for felines."

Here are a few things he routinely prescribes for diabetic canines. They are not used all at once, but incorporated gradually; thus, the list reflects what is used but not in any particular order. (The amounts indicated are for a 60-pound dog.)

> *Gymnema sylvestre* extract (in liquid or capsule form). This is a popular Ayurvedic botanical from India and is extremely useful for diabetes. Begin with one capsule three times daily and eventually increase to three capsules three times daily.
>
> A chromium supplement with pancreatic enzymes. This can be mixed into food.
>
> A manganese (10–20 mg.)–zinc (100 mg.) formula.
>
> Lecithin granules (one tablespoon) mixed with food.
>
> Flaxeed–safflower oil mixture for omega 66 fatty acids. May be mixed with food.
>
> B vitamins (two crushed tablets or one-half teaspoon brewer's yeast in food).

For a ten-pound cat, the following items have proven efficacious in the treatment of diabetes:

> *Gymnema sylvestre* fluid extract (10–20 drops given 30 minutes before each feeding session).
>
> Chromium supplement mixed in with food.
>
> A manganese (5 mg.)–zinc (25 mg.) formula.
>
> Liquid lecithin (one-half teaspoon)
>
> A vitamin E (one-half teaspoon)–cod-liver oil (one-half teaspoon) mix "for stabilization."

One nutrient I believe is extremely important in the management of animal or human diabetes is vitamin C. When most diabetic patients get blood tests, a serious deficiency in this vitamin usually shows up. Since this nutrient always enters the cells in conjunction with insulin, a deficiency of it also indicates an inefficiency in insulin activity. Small animals could use 100 mg. of vitamin C and 50 mg. of grapeseed extract or rutin to assist with its assimilation. Bigger pets would require twice or three times these amounts.

Diabetics (whether animal or human) also tend to have lower than normal blood levels of antioxidants and higher levels of free radicals and free-radical damage. Antioxidants are substances that exert a strong policing action on maverick molecules lacking electrons. Vitamin E is one of these. In the form of animal-strength wheat-germ oil, free radicals are pretty much "locked up" nutritionally and can cause no cellular havoc to speak of. Dosage requirements for small animals is one teaspoon, while larger pets get one tablespoon. (See Product Appendix under Anthropological Research Center for more on Rex Wheat Germ Oil.)

Certain herbs not only have strong antioxidant properties but also tend to be equally effective as potent hypoglycemic agents. Garlic and goldenseal root stand out from the rest in terms of these dual qualities. Some owners and veterinarians like the idea of giving raw garlic. But I don't, since there may be an untoward reaction from its oils. Therefore, I recommend that aged garlic extract from Japan be given instead: one-half teaspoon of the liquid twice daily or two capsules of the aged garlic–chromium formula opened and their contents mixed in with every meal. (See Product Appendix under Wakunga.)

Two other herbs I have used a lot in animal and human diabetes cases are kelp and dandelion root. Generally, the encapsulated powders work better for this type of problem than a tea or liquid might. I always use them together, never alone. For every two capsules of dandelion root, I include one tablet or capsule of kelp. The powdered contents can be poured directly into food. I still don't quite know why both work better together than separately. But I'm inclined to think that the iodine in the seaweed encourages the activity of the thyroid gland a little more, while the dandelion works in the liver, spleen, and pancreas as it should.

No other holistic healing book for animals or herbal reference work mentions these two in combination for diabetes treatment. It is something I formulated a number of years ago based on information given me by a coastal Salish Native American medicine man in the Northwest. It has proven of considerable merit in this disease.

One last spice should be mentioned: basil. The fresh leaves can be finely cut and included with other food intended for pet consumption. Or else one-quarter teaspoon of the powder may be substituted. Indian research has demonstrated that this delightful culinary herb can normalize blood-sugar levels and enhance the action of insulin, according to a report in the *Indian Journal of Experimental Biology* (31:891–93, 1993).

Cookies for Diabetic Dogs

I am grateful to Susan Goldstein, an animal nutritionist, for this particular recipe. Her work has been featured on two major television networks (NBC and CBS). She co-authored with her veterinarian husband, Bob, the booklet *Super Foods and Healing Meals for Pets,* from which the following was excerpted with their permission.

SUSAN'S OATMEAL COOKIES

3 cups oatmeal, uncooked

1 cup cold filtered water

1 ½ cups whole-wheat flour

1 tablespoon parsley, chopped

2 egg yolks

1 cup raisins

1 teaspoon baking soda

2 cloves garlic, shopped

Mix all ingredients together. Spoon onto a greased cookie sheet. Bake 12 to 15 minutes at 350 degrees. Place on a cooling rack. Store in refrigerator for up to two months.

DIARRHEA/DYSENTERY

Two Success Stories

Ramona Cutler of New Orleans had a five-year-old tawny-colored tabby named Cinnamon. One time it came down with an unexpected bout of diarrhea, which puzzled the owner very much. A local vet told her it could be due to any number of things and started listing some of them: worms, bacterial infection in the G.I. tract, bad food, chemical toxins, indigestible matter, emotional excitement, and so forth. The vet wanted to prescribe some metronidazole, which is standard treatment for Giardia infections, but Ramona ruled that out.

"I didn't want my kitty's system polluted with some kind of chemical drug that I didn't understand," she told me later by phone. "That's why I called you." She got my number from the back of one of my health encyclopedias.

I gave her several options from which to choose, not knowing the severity of the exact cause of the condition. She was to grate one half of an unpeeled apple and set it aside for five hours until it had turned brown. She was then to empty the contents of two capsules of Kyo-Dophilus into the apple pulp and feed a portion to her cat twice a day. If this didn't work sufficiently she was to use the same apple base, but this time add one-half teaspoon carob powder and administer the same way.

She reported back in about nine days and said that both of my suggestions worked very well. She didn't indicate if both were used at the same time or independently of each other, but vouched for their efficacy. (See the Product Appendix under Wakunaga of America for more information.)

On the other end of the country, residing in Spokane, Washington, was another young lady by the name of Tiffany Schneider. Her two-year-old Russian wolfhound came down with a mild case of dysentery. Through a friend who had purchased several of my health books in the past, she got my address and wrote, asking what could be done.

In the letter sent back I suggested a rather novel approach that I have seen used in some parts of the Orient with good success. I advised her to slowly cook on low heat for about two-and-a-half hours two-thirds cup white rice, making sure the pot was covered at all times. This was then to be set aside and cooled to lukewarm. She was to strain one cup of the rice water and add one-half teaspoon soy sauce before feeding it to her dog. She was to repeat this procedure four times daily. I also recommended adding one-half teaspoon liquid aged-garlic extract from Japan in the event there was some bacterial or viral infection. (See Product Appendix under Wakunaga for this.)

She didn't wait to write me but called the next evening to report that her dog's problem "appears to have corrected itself with the remedies you sent." She thanked me, and we both parted feeling happy to know that another animal had been made well again through natural means.

Diet Tips

Nutrition Lessons from a Tail-Wagging Convention

In the latter part of September 1997 the annual Purebred Dog Championships were held in Houston, Texas. A friend of mine who raises purebred and pedigreed English bulldogs for a living invited me to accompany him down with all my expenses paid. It was an opportunity I could ill afford to pass up. In doing so, I gained a greater understanding of where so many physical defects and body malfunctions in numerous dog breeds come from. The science of breeding canines with cute and cuddly features has resulted in dogs having more congenital malformations at birth and cats having fewer.

But enough of my soapbox opinions lest I really get carried away on something I truly feel is inhumane to domesticated house pets. While in Houston at this large show, I met Shirley McKean, who describes herself as "a professional animal dietitian." We hit it off great the first time we were introduced to each other and from there things got only better.

Shirley is one of those people who can "lecture a mile a minute." She's fully aware of being able to "talk up a storm" effortlessly and still make it appear as if she's not breathing while doing so. And what were her thoughts on diet, I wondered.

"Diet is *the* best tool, in fact, the *only* tool that a pet owner ever has with which to direct the future course of his or her animal's health. But it must begin in the puppy or kitten stage to be of any worthwhile success. *A-n-d* (she said with slow and deliberate emphasis), stay as close to natural as possible. That way you'll never stray very far from the path of good health."

She elaborated further on this last point. "Watch animals in the wild. They generally eat just *once* a day and no more. They don't have food lying in front of them all the time to tempt them with additional feedings. Young animals, of course, may need several feedings within a 24-hour period on account of their physical growth. But once they've pretty well matured, then they need to be trained to eat only one meal per day and *no more*."

By doing so, she reasoned, "you cut down the risk of that animal incurring obesity, heart disease, diabetes, kidney failure, and a host of other problems associated with overweight." Besides, "it's a lot healthier for them anyway. Animals, by nature, won't gorge themselves as people do. They eat only enough to satisfy their hunger, then walk away. Wouldn't it be great if their owners had the willpower to do that? We'd definitely have a lot less obesity in this country than we currently do."

Also, another important consideration to keep in mind: "*Don't* leave an animal's food out for longer than 30 minutes. After this, remove it; otherwise, the *smell* will tempt the animal to eat more in a little while."

And "don't fret about not feeding your dog or cat on time every day. Their ancestors in the wild have *very* irregular eating schedules, to say the least. And yet they don't starve! Pet owners need only to look at themselves and ask, 'When was the last time I ate my meals at the same time every day?' They need to give their animals a break and not be too worried if they've missed feeding Rover or Frisky by several hours. It's *no big deal*! I've known of wild dogs to go for a day or two without a meal!" Then, pausing momentarily for brief reflection, Ms. McKean added with a touch of sardonic humor, "'course, I don't know if that applies to wild cats or not. Hmm! That's probably what makes them so wild—too many hours in between their last meal."

Dietary No-Nos

Over the years Shirley has developed a rule of nutritional philosophy that "had never failed me once yet." It is this: "Garbage in, garbage out. Quality in, quality out." She then went on to explain the meaning of this. "Pet owners who are too damned lazy (her own words) to fix nutritious meals themselves for their animals and instead rely on supermarket 'junk' [which she labels as canned or packaged pet foods] are just asking for trouble in their pets down the road. Those animals in time will get sick and look scruffy on account of the chemical additives and preservatives, moldy grains, rancid fats, and spoiled meats that such foods contain. This is how I define 'garbage in, garbage out.'"

She gave her reasoning for the other adage. "If an animal is routinely fed *fresh* fruits and *organic* vegetables and *some* range-fed or contaminant-free meat, then it is going to not only feel good but also have the 'perfect look,' I inquired. "The eyes will have a luster to them; the coat will be shiny; there will be a spring or bounce in the animal's step; it will have no odor about it; the elimination cycle will always be normal; and its temperament will be fairly even and consistent," she stated.

Consumers need to be aware of labels that read *meat by-products* or *beef by-products.* In his outstanding book, *Pet Allergies: Remedies for an Epidemic* (Inglewood, CA: Very Healthy Enterprises, 1986; p. 13) (co-authored with Martin Zucker), veterinarian Alfred J. Plechner gives a more specific definition of what these two government-permitted euphemisms *actually* mean: "Diseased tissue, pus, hair, assorted slaughterhouse rejects, and carcasses in varying stages of decomposition [that have been] sterilized with chemicals, heat and pressure procedures." As awful as it may seem, the U.S. federal government allows pet-food manufacturers to obtain most of their meat or beef by-products from the industry-labeled "4-D" animals: those that are *d*ead, *d*ying, *d*iseased, and *d*isabled.

Above all, Ms. McKean insisted rather bluntly: "Pet owners should *never* trust their local vets for food recommendations." As a rule, "these people are usually trained in medical procedures and *not* nutrition." And people with pets need to read the ingredients even buying food from health-food stores. Because *not* everything in a health-food store is healthy or good for you!" I gave a hearty "amen" to that statement.

I asked for her thoughts on something I've recommended through the years for people and have carried over to pets. I told her about my "50/50 Diet" in which 50 percent (or thereabouts) of the diet consisted of good, solid nutritious substances and the balance (or close thereto) was store-bought, packaged, and refined foods. I said, "This isn't the optimal diet by any means. But it certainly is more affordable and realistic for the economic and busy times we live in than a 100-percent all-natural and totally organic diet." After a minute's pause pondering, she said, "Sure, why not? You're right . . . it isn't the ideal by any means, but what the heck . . . you gotta start somewhere, and I guess this is as good a place as any to begin if you can't afford or don't have time for the other. At the very least, an animal gets the benefit of *some* good food."

"Half a loaf is better than no loaf," I philosophized. "And if people will vary the foods from both ends of the spectrum and make sure that they and their pets get *some* nutritious staples in them *every* day, along with a little of the not-so-good food, then their bodies will have a fighting chance to somehow make it and remain relatively healthy."

Something Fishy about Tuna

We compared notes on tuna fish, one of the most common *flavoring* ingredients in cat food. Essentially, canned tuna has two drawbacks, as we saw it. First, the vegetable oil it's packed in tends to rob the feline of vitamin E. Second, tuna ranks high on the list for mercury content. (A favorite joke of mine through the years has been that with so much mercury in a can of tuna, you can hang it outside the window on a string and use it as a crude thermometer if you don't have the real thing.) Much of the tuna used in cat food comes from the red-meat part of the fish, which contains considerably more toxins than the white-meat tuna that humans regularly consume.

Cats become easily "hooked" on tuna just as people do on "crack cocaine." Some veterinarians describe a feline so hooked as being a "tuna junkie." Manufacturers, knowing the great power that tuna holds over such animals, include it in most of their cat foods so as to have felines form an attraction for their particular brands.

Shirley and I then discussed what fish might be more appropriate for cats than tuna. We came up with canned salmon, mackerel, and sardines, as well as fresh-water fish such as rainbow trout that had been steamed or baked as having the least amount of mercury in them. (Some salt-water fish are also acceptable.)

Making Your Dog into a Vegetarian

I interrupt my narrative with Shirley McKean to pursue another line of thought regarding a dog's feeding habits. Recently, in a long-distance telephone conversation with Diana Petersen of St. Albert, Alberta, Canada (close to Edmonton), I learned that "it is easier to turn your dog into a vegetarian than it is with a cat." "Cats, by nature," she noted, "are meat-eaters and have had meat-eating instincts genetically bred into them over thousands of years."

Mrs. Petersen and her husband have two purebred rottweilers that are two-and-a-half years of age: a male named Foli and his female companion, Wyllo. The couple also have some three-year-old cats of Persian mix: a tom named Jasper and a feline named Kandey.

"The secret to getting dogs to liking vegetables," she said, "is to always flavor whatever they're eating, whether raw or cooked, with a little beef or *fish* broth." This remark astonished me enough to comment that "I didn't know dogs liked fish." "Oh yes, very much so," she added. "They go crazy over mackerel or sardine oil or a little salmon or pike broth poured over their veggies.

"They like just about anything in the vegetable line. You name it, and they probably like it: carrots, asparagus, kale, potatoes, celery, even lettuce sometimes. I'll either cook or grate most of these items, but always bake the potatoes. I've even juiced some of these things, such as mixing carrot juice with a little juice from celery, parsley, or lettuce. I then flavor it with a little beef or fish broth and they just lap it up.

"And when I give them dry food morning and night, I always add just a small amount of either broth. Not too much, though, or the food becomes soggy and they won't enjoy it as much. We like to feed them Shaklee's Addition. I give them four cups in the morning and again at night; they clean everything up. To every four cups of dry food, I will add between one-half and three-quarters cup of broth and mix it in good with the other."

Mrs. Petersen also makes a vegetable puree out of leftovers from the dinner table. "Both our dogs and cats really take to this," she remarked, provided she has added a touch of meat broth or oil to it. "Getting your dogs used to a vegetarian diet takes some time, patience, and gentle persuasion. It isn't something you accomplish in a week or even a month. There is a psychological strategy at work here. You must do it with love and understanding . . . *and* a little bribery." That's where the meat broths and fish oils come into play.

Her son finished a two-year mission for The Church of Jesus Christ of Latter-Day Saints in the Utah Salt Lake City Mission, where he eventually met me. I gave him one of my health encyclopedias which he mailed home to his mom, whom I contacted for the interview for this book.

Pet Supplementation

The 1998 Purebred Dog Championships show in Houston came off fairly orderly, but was still a tad noisy for both Ms. McKean and me. So she, the animal dietitian, and I moved to quieter quarters where we continued our lengthy conversation on nutrition-related topics. She gave me two vitamin-mineral formulas intended to meet the nutritional needs of puppies and kittens. They follow here.

PUPPY NUTRITIONAL MIX

This mixture should be made ahead of time and kept in the refrigerator. It can be sprinkled over food: 1¼ teaspoons for puppies up to 6 pounds; 2½ teaspoons for 6 to 16 pounds; 3¼ teaspoons for 17–39 pounds; 2½ tablespoons for 40–59 pounds; 3¾ tablespoons for 60 to 89 pounds; and ⅔ cup for dogs over 90 pounds. Put in the food supply every day.

2 cups food yeast
2 cups brewer's yeast

(continued)

½ cup kelp powder

½ cup beet-root-juice powder

½ cup barley powder

½ cup lecithin granules

1 ½ cups wheat bran

1 ½ cups bonemeal, calcium lactate, or calcium gluconate

Mix all of these dry ingredients together in a bread machine or by hand. Besides this, a puppy needs daily allotments of vitamin C. Use the pediatric drops intended for children. Newly weaned puppies should get no more than 30 mg., while 4-month-old puppies should receive about 150 mg. Those older than 4 months of age could do with 600–750 mg. per day. *Note:* Keep vitamin C separate from formula mix.

KITTEN NUTRITIONAL MIX

Prepare and refrigerate the same as that for puppies.

Sprinkle one-quarter teaspoon in food for kittens and triple this amount for a mature feline every day.

¼ cup food yeast

¼ cup brewer's yeast

¼ cup wheat bran

¼ cup kelp powder

¼ cup beet-root-juice powder

¼ cup barley powder

¼ cup lecithin granules

¼ cup bonemeal, calcium lactate, or calcium gluconate.

Thoroughly mix all of the dry ingredients. (Consult the Product Appendix under Pines as a potential source for obtaining the beet-juice and barley powders. The rest of the items may be obtained from a local health-food store, with the exception of the food yeast, which may have to come from a supermarket.)

In addition, use children's vitamin C drops but, as with the instructions previously given under the puppy formula, *do not mix* the two of them together, but always administer separately.

It is also important to give your puppy or kitten, as well as your mature dog or cat, one teaspoon of Rex Wheat Germ Oil, which is specifically intended for animals (although many humans take it as well with good results). (See the Product Appendix under Anthropological Research Center for information on obtaining this.)

Yummy Recipes for Young Animals

After a couple of hours of chatting on the first day of the dog-championship convention, we met again the following afternoon to continue our dialogue. She volunteered a couple of recipes that "will provide balanced nourishment for newborn and young pets." Ms. McKean noted that "both recipes provide a basic framework within which the pet owner can experiment to create his or her recipes," if need be. After all, healthy creativity is what meal diversification is all about. And in this respect, animals are really no different from us: They like variety in much the same way we do.

DO-IT-YOURSELF PUPPY MEAL

1 pound ground turkey or *ground beef* or *fish; browned well, drained of most fat but not all of it*

2 eggs, scrambled or hard-boiled

1 medium potato; cooked and mashed, including the skin; or use cooked rice or tofu at other times

½ cup cooked oatmeal or *cooked cracked barley*

1 cup black beans, cooked, mashed

¼ cup grated carrots

¼ cup finely grated raw vegetables (broccoli, spinach, green beans)

2 tablespoons cold-pressed flaxseed oil or *extra-virgin olive oil*

3 tablespoons liquid aged garlic extract from Japan*

1 tablespoons barley powder*

1 tablespoon blackstrap molasses

*See the Product Appendix under Wakunaga and Pines respectively.

(continued)

Put everything in a large plastic bowl and mix well. For a puppy five pounds or under, divide into four equal portions that will last four days. For a puppy over five pounds, divide into two equal portions for two days. Serve a small portion three times a day. Seal the bowl with a tight-fitting lid and refrigerate.

With each serving, Ms. McKean advised that a pet owner add some of her Puppy Nutritional Mix.

Do-It-Yourself Kitten Meal

1 pound ground chicken or *ground beef, browned well, drained of most fat but not all of it*

¾ cup canned mackerel or *½ cup sardines*

4 ounces tofu or *grated cheddar cheese*

2 eggs, scrambled or hard-boiled

2 cups wild rice, cooked, or *1 ½ cups cooked oatmeal flavored with a little fish broth or fish oil*

1 cup cooked black beans, mashed

¼ cup grated carrots or *asparagus* or *other grated raw vegetables*

1 tablespoon extra-virgin olive oil

1 teaspoon safflower oil

1 ½ teaspoons liquid aged-garlic extract from Japan*

½ teaspoon beet-root-juice powder*

1 tablespoon blackstrap molasses or *sorghum*

*See the Product Appendix under Wakunaga and Pines respectively.

Follow the same procedures for mixing and feeding as those given with the puppy meal. Except here portion dividing is governed not by weight but rather by the age of the kitten. For kittens four months and under, divide into ten equal portions which will last ten days. For kittens four months and older, divide into seven equal portions, which will last a week.

And don't forget to add a little Kitten Nutritional Mix to each meal.

Wholesome Nourishment for Mature Dogs and Cats

The final recipe that Ms. McKean happily provided is intended for adult pets. She stated, "This recipe relies on organically raised, fresh food whenever possible and is very nourishing to dogs and cats."

DO-IT-YOURSELF MATURE PET MEAL

16 ounces fresh ground lamb or duck or turkey (make sure all bones are removed)

7 ounces spring water with 5 drops liquid ConcenTrace*

9 ounces cooked old-fashioned oats (just ⅓ of this, or 3 ounces, for cats)

9 ounces pureed zucchini, carrots, broccoli, cauliflower, artichoke hearts, or alfalfa sprouts (just ⅓ of this, or 3 ounces, for cats)

1 tablespoon beet-juice powder*

1 tablespoon barley powder*

1 teaspoon liquid aged-garlic extract from Japan*

1 teaspoon cold-pressed flaxseed oil

1 teaspoon cod-liver oil

1 teaspoon Rex Wheat Germ Oil*

*Consult the Product Appendix under Trace Minerals Research, Pines, Wakunaga, and Anthropological Research Center for obtaining each ingredient with an asterisk by it.

Blend everything together in a blender to the consistency of thick porridge or chili. Refrigerate for three days; it can also be frozen for one-half year.

Protein: Overload or Under Limit?

In the final phase of our two-day discussion, Ms. McKean and I spoke about pet protein needs. She mentioned seeing "a large number of household pets being fed nearly all-meat diets" by well-meaning owners. The results, though, are anything but good for the poor animals. "They're usually in some degree of poor health, showing skin inflammation, diarrhea, and odor. The first thing I do is to cut their protein overload by 90 percent. Then we start seeing signs of improvement within days: Their coats become glossy; they're much more energetic and a lot happier."

We both agreed that household animals need more fiber in their diets. Fiber is a sure guarantee for intestinal health. Additional fiber in the diet will also keep a dog or cat from becoming obese. Fiber helps to control diabetes by regulating blood-sugar levels in normally healthy pets.

Animals need certain vitamins and minerals just as we do. We both placed vitamins A, C and E high on our lists. Vitamin A can come from cod-liver or some other type of fish oil, as well as leafy green vegetables and carrots (in the beta-carotene form). Vitamin C is always necessary to ward off infection. This should preferably be given in liquid or powdered form and mixed in with food. Ms. McKean was familiar with Rex Wheat Germ Oil and agreed that it was the best source of vitamin E around; one teaspoon for cats and smaller dogs and one tablespoon for larger animals every *other* day, we believed would be sufficient. (See Product Appendix under Anthropological Research Center.)

However, we differed on our sources for an animal's mineral needs. Ms. McKean thought that bonemeal was adequate for calcium. I, on the other hand, preferred liquid ionic minerals from the Great Salt Lake in the form of ConcenTrace. (See Product Appendix under Trace Minerals Research.) Powdered seaweeds such as dulse, kelp, or bladderwrack were good sources for iodine. And dark leafy greens such as powdered stinging nettle or powdered or finely minced parsley were excellent for iron. We both claimed alfalfa as an all-around vegetable source for most mineral needs. In addition to this, I added wheat or barley grass to the list, which she didn't. (See Product Appendix under Pines.)

Our conversation soon swung back to the subject of protein. We both concurred that the most ideal protein for a pet was an egg white. A close second was soybean (preferably in milk and tofu forms). We differed somewhat on the number of meaty meals to be served during typical week-long feedings. I felt that five days of some meat (with fresh or lightly cooked vegetables and cooked grains included) was essential for cats, since they are true carnivores. She believed that felines required some meat every single day. But, we found agreement when it came to dogs: they're much easier to make into vegetarians, or at least *semi*-vegetarians, which I think is more prudent, given their carnivorous nature.

Finally, we expressed a common belief that pet owners should be concerned as much with the quality of what they give their animals as with the quantity. I went to Houston with a buddy and came away with a new friendship and a great deal of information that soon proved useful in this project. And who says that purebred dog shows aren't exciting and worthwhile?

A Third Opinion

Given that many animal-care authorities have widely differing opinions on what may or may not be good for pets, it is always good to get a second or even a third opinion in matters of great importance. Whether or not a dog should be gradually introduced to a total or semi-vegetarian diet is one of these. In the preceding paragraphs, two such opinions were given. Shirley McKean, the animal dietitian, was for *complete* vegetarianism in canines. My approach, on the other hand, was more practical and realistic: I opted for a diet that was only *semi*-vegetarian, with quality meat occasionally served.

For some dog owners, however, there may be a third alternative: *no* vegetarianism, period. I am grateful to Laura Williams of Milan, Illinois, for sharing the following true ordeal that she went through as an owner of several dogs from 1989 to 1995. I will let her tell her own unhappy story, which should make owners think twice and get considerable advice from different veterinarians before attempting to turn their own canines into "veggie dogs" for life.

"I had become a vegetarian because of animal rights and later learned of all the health benefits of being a vegetarian. I'm sure like a few other vegetarians out there, I debated over feeding my companion animals meat, and I wanted all those health benefits for my 'kids.' So in 1989, I began feeding by two dogs, Blacki and Sheiba, a homemade vegetarian diet—what could be better, natural food, right? In 1991, I adopted Tyler and began him on a homemade vegetarian diet also. In 1991, Blacki died of heart failure, believed to be, but not properly diagnosed as dilated cardiomyopathy (DCM). Otherwise, they did extremely well on the diet, displaying energy, wonderful coats, health, and vigor, and never seeing a vet for anything other than the normal physical checkup.

"In 1994, Tyler was diagnosed with DCM and six months later he died, along with a part of me. Before Tyler died, I called my vegetarian dog-food supplier to check on the potassium and salt content in the diet. He told me Tyler probably wouldn't have lived this long if it weren't for his vegetarian diet. I was surprised to learn that he was aware of taurine and carnitine deficiencies in the diet that has been known to cause DCM in dogs and that employees of 'an animal-rights group that advocated vegetarian diets for companion animals' were giving their dogs carnitine supplements. How could these people suspect this and not even tell the owners of vegetarian dogs?

"After learning this, I suspected my other two dogs might also have DCM, although they showed no clinical signs. In December, my fear was confirmed. I not only caused Tyler's death, I also caused my other two dogs to develop DCM (by placing them on a vegetarian diet). I feared that the disease may have progressed too far to be irreversible. My veterinarian placed them on taurine supplements and changed their diet. Three weeks later, Molli was fine, no DCM. Sheiba had also improved, but wasn't out of it totally. I mourn Tyler's loss, though, knowing I won't be able to see him again, at least not in this life.

"I urge anyone who has a veggie dog to get an ultrasound for that pet. Don't rely on clinical signs or X-rays and EKGs alone. I don't want anyone to go through the guilt and despair I'm going through, and I don't want my dogs to die of DCM because of their diets ever again!"

DISTEMPER (CANINE AND FELINE)

Canine: a Progressive Disease

Most dogs become exposed to the canine distemper virus at some point in their lives, since it is airborne. But they can also pick it up from contaminated food or water dishes, plastic toys, and discarded bones. If their immune systems are strong enough, however, they can usually withstand the virus.

The first sign of infection, though, for those unlucky enough to get it, is a fever three to six days later. The animal usually recovers and appears to be doing well for almost a week before the second wave of symptoms hit: another fever, clear discharges from the eyes and nose, and no desire to eat. Shortly thereafter symptoms become more intense as the problem advances to a new level: extremely bad conjunctivitis of the eyes and eyelids; considerable mucus discharge from the nose; foul-smelling diarrhea; the appearance of rash or sores on the belly or in the anal area.

Other evident signs seen in some but not all cases include depression, seizures, muscle incoordination, muscle tremors, and slight paralysis.

Finding Solutions that Work

Richard Pitcairn, DVM, who switched his practice to more holistic methods, declares in his book, *Dr. Pitcairn's Complete Guide to Natural Health for Dogs & Cats* (Emmaus, PA: Rodale Press, Inc., 1995; p. 257), "Though I have treated many distemper cases with the orthodox approach of antibiotics, fluids, and other drugs, I have not seen it do much good." Another veterinarian in the Southwest confided that he "doesn't place much faith in the standard veterinary medications for this kind of problem," believing instead that "nutrition is the best approach to solving it safely."

A mild food fast must be imposed on the sick animal during the acute phase of this disease. *No meat* or other solids should be given. Instead, offer the sick canine *fresh* vegetable juices every day. These are rich in mineral salts and will help to evacuate poisons from the dog's system in order to make it well again. They will also give the animal strength during its weakened physical state.

The machine I recommend for this is a Vita-Mix 5000. It is the only juicer I know of that includes the fiber with the juice. This is important since the fiber of fruits and vegetables contain many valuable nutrients that would otherwise never be assimilated were the fiber to be discarded. (See the Product Appendix under Vita-Mix for more information on this fine machine.)

Tokyo Dog, Teriyaki Style

1 cup chopped tomatoes
½ cup celery with leaves
2 tablespoons sweet green bell pepper
4 baby carrots
2 tablespoons raw onion
2 tablespoons Teriyaki Sauce
1 ½ cups ice cubes

Place all of the ingredients in the Vita-Mix 5000 in the order given. Secure the two-part lid by locking under its tabs. Move the black speed control to the HIGH position. Lift the black lever to the ON position and permit the unit to run almost 2 minutes, until the contents are smooth. Let the liquid set at room temperature for 20 minutes before pouring into the dog's feeding bowl. Makes 3 cups.

Boxer Rebellion

1 cup fresh tomatoes
½ cup lettuce
¼ cup carrots
1 tablespoon onion
3 sprigs parsley
¼ cup sweet red- or green-bell pepper
¼ teaspoon Worcestershire sauce
pinch of granulated kelp (a seaweed)
1 cup ice cubes

Place all of these ingredients in the Vita-Mix 5000 in the order given. Secure the lid as suggested in the previous recipe. Move the different levers to the positions previously indicated. Run the unit for one-and-one-half minutes until everything is well mixed and has a smooth consistency. Set aside for 20 minutes until some of the chill has disappeared, then serve to your canine friend. Makes about one-and-three-quarters cups.

You can also make various vegetable broths by adding one cup of chopped vegetables (broccoli, cabbage, carrots, kale, potatoes, turnips) with one cup boiling water and one chicken or beef bouillon cube (for flavoring) to the Vita-Mix 5000 container and mixing everything together for one-and-one-half minutes. Small animals find this very tasty.

A dog can go for up to ten days without solid food before signs of starvation become evident. For most canines a period less than this is adequate. Pure water (other than from the tap) should always be made available.

Some nutritional supplements may be necessary besides the daily allotment of fresh juices or warm vegetable broth. Vitamin C in liquid form is helpful for rebuilding the immune system and increasing resistance to viral infection. I suggest 1,000 mg. daily, divided into four increments of 250 mg. each. This can be added to the dog's juice, broth, or drinking water.

In cases of extreme conjunctivitis, special attention needs to be paid to the eyes and eyelids of an animal with distemper. A solution I've often used in the past for such conditions calls for pouring one-and-a-half cups of boiling distilled water over one-half teaspoon of wild Oregon grape or goldenseal-root powder. The mixture is thoroughly stirred with a spoon, covered, and permitted to set for 20 minutes. The liquid is then strained through a clean piece of cotton cloth or unused coffee-filter paper. One-quarter teaspoon of boric acid powder is then added to the new container and the contents vigorously shaken. (The herbs may be purchased at any health-food store. The distilled water is available at any supermarket, and the boric acid may be found in any pharmacy.)

Each time the dog's eyes are to be bathed with this solution, only a little bit should be poured out into a small clean dish. The rest should be set aside in the cupboard, where it will keep for several days. Use Q-tips soaked in the solution to remove thickened mucus from the eyes and eyelids. Discard any liquid left over rather than returning it to the original batch.

Pour out a tiny amount of extra-virgin olive oil from its bottle onto a clean plate. Dip a Q-tip in the oil and gently lubricate the rim of each eye and around the eyelids. This will provide healing and reduce dryness.

Homeopathic medicine is popular with a number of holistic-minded veterinarians, and they don't hesitate to use some of the drugs common to this treatment. However, as cited elsewhere in the text, in good conscience I cannot recommend it to humans or animals. This, of course, is strictly my own opinion and readers can use their own intelligence to evaluate pros and cons of homeopathy for themselves.

Canine distemper is an aggressive infection that can leave a dog's nervous, digestive, and physical systems considerably weakened from the ordeal. I recommend feeding such an animal the cooled liquid from boiled oats, to which has been added some Kyolic liquid aged-garlic extract from Japan. To one-half cup regular oats add six cups of distilled or pure water and boil, uncovered, for 20 minutes. Strain through a wire sieve and set aside to cool. With each cup of oat water, add six drops of Kyolic liquid (see the Product Appendix under Wakunaga of America). Give this to the dog at least twice a day, morning and evening. This is wonderful nourishment and will enable the pet to gradually regain its strength.

Feline: a Disease by Several Names

In contacting several different veterinarians with regard to the feline side of this infection I discovered that it went by various names, depending on whom I was speaking with at the time. A Colorado doctor referred to it simply as "cat distemper," while his colleague from New Mexico labeled it "cat chorea." (This term, I later learned from others, is actually an effect of the actual viral infection itself and involves continual twitching of a cat's leg, hip, or shoulder muscles.)

A Los Angeles County veterinarian used the terms "feline distemper" and "infectious enteritis" interchangeably as he spoke with me about this common condition, which comes on quickly and without much advance notice. A Boston veterinary clinic took the high literary road, calling the disease by its proper medical name: feline panleukopenia—all of which goes to show that for some ailments there can be a multiplicity of terms to describe them.

What to Look for

An infected cat generally assumes what is considered to be a typical "panleukopenia posture": its sternum and chin rest on the floor, feet are tucked beneath the body, and the top of the shoulder blades are elevated above the back. Dehydration comes quickly, and the feline will prefer to rest its head on the edge of the water dish in order to lap up badly needed liquid every so often. It isn't uncommon for a sick animal to evacuate its stomach contents into its water or food dish.

Fever is inevitable and is generally mild to moderate in the early stages of the disease. But body temperature can drastically escalate as the cat's condition becomes extremely grave. Occasionally there is abdominal pain, and the small intestine may even feel a little loose or lax.

Obviously, when an animal isn't feeling in top shape, its mental state is adversely affected. The worse the physical symptoms are, so, too, will be a feline's emotions. Depression isn't a condition relegated solely to humans, but makes an equal impact on sick animals. And since cats, in particular, are especially sensitive, their depression would be expected to be of greater magnitude than that experienced by a sick dog. So more than just correct diet and natural remedies should be at work here in helping a cat get over its distemper: The animal should be gently stroked with the fingers and talked to as much as the owner's time will allow. Bolstering the confidence of a sick pet reassures the animal that it is still loved in spite of not being well. Too often owners forget this social dimension as they seek other ways to improve the physical health of their ailing pets.

Recovery Treatments

In his book on natural pet care, Dr. Pitcairn has this to say about treatment procedures for cat distemper: "The most crucial factor in successful treatment is to catch the disorder in its earliest stages. Since young animals can die very quickly, there often isn't enough time to get a home treatment under way." Because distemper can be more rapid and fatal in cats than in dogs, time is of the essence in quickly dealing with the problem in an effective manner.

The "Three D's" (as I call them) of feline panleukopenia are *dehydration*, *depression*, and *diarrhea*. One herb will easily solve all three problems at once. This is catnip. Bring one pint of distilled or pure water to a boil. Stir in two tablespoons of cut, dried herb and leaves. Cover with a lid and set aside to steep for 30 minutes. Strain half the liquid and put in the cat's water dish instead of regular water. The remaining tea will keep for 48 hours at room temperature. About every third day make a fresh batch and discard the old.

I've used catnip tea with great success in feline distemper. A cat may not drink as much of the tea as it might plain water, but the herb will adequately meet the animal's fluid needs. The nepetalactones contained in catnip exert a positive influence on the cat's brain, creating a happier mood in the animal. These nepetalactones also exhibit certain disinfectant and antispasmodic properties which help counteract viral-induced diarrhea.

Some veterinarians recommend that vitamin C be given every few hours: 100 mg. to very young kittens and double this amount to young and adult cats. Dr. Pitcairn advised giving this nutrient in the form of sodium ascorbate powder mixed with water. I prefer the liquid form of vitamin C. An Arizona animal-supply company offers a more concentrated vitamin-C powder (one-half teaspoon equals 2,000 mg.) which can be mixed into food for finicky eaters. (See Holistic Animal Care in the Product Appendix.)

Feline distemper moves quickly through a cat's body and often can prove fatal. If a cat appears to be in a comatose state, there will be little or no movement in its paws, ears, and tail (those areas manifesting the greatest amount of physical expression). Its nose will have acquired a blue or purple hue. A small dab of tea-tree oil, eucalyptus oil, peppermint oil, or even camphor on a cotton ball and held in front of the cat's nose for no longer than 30 seconds at a time should be enough to revive the animal. Gently prying its mouth open and squirting 6 to 8 drops of fluid extract of cayenne down its throat will reanimate the creature further. A rectal thermometer carefully inserted into the anus will give a true reading of body temperature (about 100° F. or less) to show that most of the fever danger is past and that the animal can now be fed more solid foods.

There are several nourishing drinks that a cat can be given during its initial period of illness. I recommend a unit such as the Vita-Mix 5000 for making them instead of just any ordinary blender. (See the Product Appendix under Vita-Mix Corp. for more information.)

SIAMESE SOUP MIX

½ cup frozen peas, thawed
1-inch slice sweet red-bell pepper
2-inch slice carrot
¼ cup onion
1 cup boiling fish stock
6 drops liquid Kyolic aged-garlic extract*
3 drops ConcenTrace*

*See the Product Appendix under Wakunaga of America and Trace Minerals Research, respectively.

This mix will yield approximately 2 cups. Divide into four feeding portions over a 36-hour period.

MEOW TODDY, VEGETARIAN STYLE

1 cup spinach
¼ cup onion
1 tablespoon Pines Wheat Grass*
1 tablespoon dry powdered milk
1 chicken or fish bouillon cube
pinch of granulated kelp (a seaweed)
5 drops liquid Kyolic aged-garlic extract*
1 cup water, boiling

*See Product Appendix under Pines International and Wakunaga of America, respectively.

This recipe makes two cups. This can be divided into four equal servings spread over 36 to 48 hours. Refrigerate the amount that isn't used and reheat it to lukewarm before serving.

Two other things that cats like a lot and that can be used to help a sick feline regain its strength are sardines and liver. A small amount of either, mixed in with either soup recipe and offered to an ailing cat, will have a remarkable tonifying effect upon its system. In no time at all, pussy will be back on its feet and as lively as ever.

For mucus discharge from the eyes or nose, follow the simple instructions already given under canine distemper. With plenty of rest, lots of liquids, adequate nourishment, and sufficient care and attention, even the sickest dog or cat will somehow manage to revive at the last possible moment. All it needs is someone who loves the animal enough to give it a will to continue living.

(Also see under Anorexia for further information.)

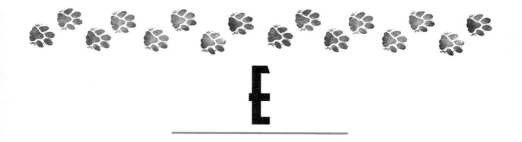

E

EAR DISCHARGES

It's All in the Ears

An animal's ears are subject to any number of different problems. These may range from excess wax secretions to tiny ear mites. Unlike human ears, those belonging to a cat or dog are for more than just hearing sounds. They tend to form part of the pet's character and signal particular moods it may be in. No two pairs of dog ears are alike. Those of a cocker spaniel denote affection, while the ears belonging to a German shepherd signify vigilance and readiness. And the temperament of any cat can be easily determined by looking at which position its ears are resting.

Television and movie actor Leonard Nimoy, who played the Vulcan named Spock on the popular hit series *Star Trek,* was once asked a most peculiar kind of question by a fan at a science-fiction convention celebrating the show. "If Spock had owned a dog, what would the shape of *its* ears have been?" (For those unacquainted with this sci/fi program, Spock had *pointed* ears.) Nimoy rubbed his chin in thoughtful contemplation and then responded, "Probably *pointed* just like his master's." Then with a mischievous grin, he added, "In that case, I guess a lot of dogs here on earth probably have some Vulcan genes in them" (referring, of course, to *their* pointed ears).

A Lesson in Dog Care at Radio City Music Hall

You never know what to expect in life. Information that at the moment may not be needed can sometimes come from the most unlikely sources and at the least opportune moments. If one is wise the unanticipated data are recorded for possible reference in the distant future. Otherwise, if a person acts carelessly and without regard, snippets of knowledge that briefly appear may be forever lost afterwards.

It was almost two decades ago, in January 1981, when I was in New York City with some friends to attend a one-of-a-kind film event. My hosts and I, along with 6,000 other patrons, were packed into Radio City Music Hall like so many sardines for the special showing of the 50-year-old four-hour silent film about Napoleon Bonaparte.

During several much appreciated intermissions, the Radio City lobby buzzed with excitement as theatergoers marveled at the film's evergreen impact.

I was standing off to one side with a cup of soda in my hand paying attention to no one in particular when I overheard part of an ongoing conversation between two women. Both were decked out in some obvious elegance and had affluent airs about them. The one was telling the other what she did for her poor dog, Mitzy (the breed was never specified).

Since herbs were part of that discussion, I set my drink down and moved in a little closer to hear them better. I scribbled highlights of the rest of their conversation on the back of an extra program I had folded and put in the inside pocket of my jacket. The discussion went something like this:

First Woman: Mitzy's ears were too oily. So what I did was warm up a tiny amount of almond oil I got from the Vitamin Cottage [a now-defunct Manhattan health-food store]. I prewarmed it in a small wine glass that I set in a bigger container half-filled with hot water.

Second Woman: And then?

First Woman: I'm getting there. I had my hubby assist me. He held Mitzy's head sideways and lifted up one ear flap at a time, while I put some of this warm oil inside her ear with an eyedropper. Then I massaged the ear canal from the outside with my fingers positioned at the base of the ear opening. This loosened up much of her accumulated ear wax. I dabbed away some of the excess oil with a few pieces of tissue paper. Harold [her husband] then turned Mitzy's head the other way for the same treatment. This prevented my dog from shaking her head and getting oil all over our beautiful carpets.

Second Woman: Imagine that, will you!

First Woman: How's your little Darla doing?

Second Woman: Oh, thanks for asking. She's getting along in years, but our vet says she still has quite a bit of spunk and life left in her.

First Woman: How old is she now?

Second Woman: She turned 14 a week ago. For her birthday treat, I took her to a famous animal psychic, who read her paws and told us her fortune.

First Woman: You don't say!

Second Woman: Darla had a strange discharge from one of her ears a while back. It had a peculiar smell to it, so I took her to that doctor in midtown…oh, what's his name?. . . Anyway, he put some aloe-vera solution into the ear from a tiny plastic squeeze bottle and told me to keep doing that twice a day until it stopped.

First Woman: And did it work?

Second Woman: Oh, heavens yes!

About this time the second intermission was winding down and everyone started moving back into the main hall. I put away my notes and enjoyed the rest of *Napoleon,* which in its original form had been an anguishing nine-and-a-half hours long. I later finished filling in from memory the rest of this most enlightening conversation between two ladies of some social distinction in regard to their cherished pets.

EPILEPSY

A "Grab Bag" of Other Problems

It appears that epilepsy may be a catch-all for a variety of different problems. At least that was the thinking of half a dozen or so veterinarians whom I spoke with by telephone in five Western states. One Oklahoma doctor pointed to hypoglycemia or low blood sugar as being a leading factor in animal convulsions. A veterinarian practicing out of the Texas Panhandle was of the opinion that worms or even chemical toxins might be partly responsible. A New Mexico vet noted that other diseases such as distemper or a head injury could produce seizures.

Epilepsy occurs with greater frequency in dogs than it does in cats. Tracking the source for it, though, is a difficult job even for the most experienced vet to do. As a Colorado doctor explained, "It really is a 'grab-bag' or oddball mixture of other contributing problems. Seldom do I ever see a seizure case that isn't based on other things."

Nutrition Is the Key to Seizure Control

It is important that the afflicted animal's brain gets the proper nourishment and nutrition it needs. This means adequate blood flow and a blood supply that is nutrient-rich in those particular elements that will help to control present and prevent future seizures from happening.

Sulfur is one of these. In another book, *Dr. Heinerman's Encyclopedia of Nature's Vitamins & Minerals* (Paramus, NJ: Prentice Hall, 1998; p. 351), I explain how a protein-modifying form of this mineral known as methylsulfonylmethane (MSM) assists the body in a number of different ways, including nerve and muscle problems that seem to be the case in the brain so far as epilepsy goes.

Recently, I interviewed two women from Colorado in my research center in Salt Lake City, one of whom had had an experience in curing her own dog of seizures by giving it MSM. The woman's name is B. G. Lundin, and she resides in the small town of Divide, located about 35 miles west of Colorado Springs. Here is her story:

I have a Chesapeake Bay retriever who developed seizures at the age of eight. Her name is Cassie. My dog would become dizzy for no apparent reason at all. She would then topple over on her side and commence trembling and going into a classic seizure mode. Because this was occurring 30 to 40 times every day, it became of great concern to me.

At that time I lived near Madison, Wisconsin. I took Cassie to the University of Wisconsin College of Veterinary Medicine, where she was examined by several very competent vets. They ran a number of tests but could give no logical explanation for these seizures. They were reluctant to prescribe any medications because they didn't know exactly what to attribute the problem to. So I took her back home.

A friend of mine in Colorado by the name of Roy Davis recommended that I try using some MSM on her. I emptied three 500 mg. capsules (or the equivalent of one-quarter teaspoon) into her food twice a day. Within days I could see the effects immediately. The number of seizure fits dropped off dramatically in my dog. Within a week's time she was experiencing no more of them. I was overjoyed and unable to fully express my gratitude to the man who had told me about MSM. I kept Cassie on this mineral supplement for the next two years until she finally passed away of old age. During that period she again experienced a full life of swimming and romping around as all normal and healthy dogs ought to be doing.

See Product Appendix under Total Life International for more on MSM. Also look under Upper Respiratory Infections for another remarkable case in which methylsulfonylmethane was efficacious in healing a kitten of lung problems.

Other equally important nutrients are a complete B complex— use 25 mg. of B per day in your pet's food. Supplement this with three-quarters teaspoon of lecithin granules and 15 mg. of zinc gluconate. You may have to break off a small section of a single B-complex tablet and a zinc tablet, then crush them into powder before mixing in the animal's food. Also give 400 mg. of vitamin C per day.

Since I don't believe in giving any animals homeopathic preparations, I will forgo mentioning anything about this further. But look under the section marked Paralysis to see how the herb bilberry may be used along with MSM, B complex, zinc, and vitamin C with good results for this and other neurological problems. Empty two capsules of powdered bilberry into the pet's food, which will greatly assist in the delivery of all nutrients to the brain more quickly. (Consult the Product Appendix under Scandinavian Naturals for information on their bilberry extract.)

EYE DISORDERS

The Amazing Benefits of Bilberry

Those who are acquainted with the healing virtues of this particular herbal fruit know that it is exceptional in the treatment of different eye problems. During the Second World War, British aviators were given rations of bilberry jam before night flying to improve their visual acuity. This is *fact* and not folklore.

Bilberry is a rich source of antioxidants. These are nutrients that manifest a policing action on free radicals, scavenger molecules that create biochemical havoc at a cellular level. The strongest of these is anthocyanin, a flavonoid of a blue-red pigment that gives the berry its deep royal-blue color and contributes to the unique flavor. A great deal of research has been done in Europe with it. Bilberry extracts (Strix) are used therapeutically to enhance collagen and lower blood pressure behind the eyeball. This helps to stave off some of the bad effects usually associated with diabetic retinopathy, retinitis pigmentosa, macular degeneration and hemorrhagic retinopathy, not to mention halting the progression of senile cortical cataracts. (Consult the Product Appendix under Scandinavian Naturals for Strix.)

These are human conditions, but a few, such as cataracts or corneal ulcers, also occur in dogs and cats. The favorite remedy for some veterinarians in the United Kingdom is to mix one teaspoon each of the fluid extracts of bilberry and eyebright herb together with one teaspoon of cod-liver oil. This is then mixed in with the animal's food twice a day. (Double this amount should be used for larger-sized dogs such as Dobermans or Saint Bernards.)

Eye problems may also be treated with a tea made from celandine or chickweed herb or mallow flowers or the leaves of sage or yellow dock. Any one of these makes a wonderfully soothing remedy for eye inflammation. Boil one pint of distilled or spring water; add one teaspoon of any herb; stir, cover, and set aside to steep for 30 minutes. Strain and bathe the animal's eyes several times daily with this infusion.

(The reader is encouraged to consult other entries within the text that have to do with eye problems: Conjunctivitis, Infection, and Red Eye.)

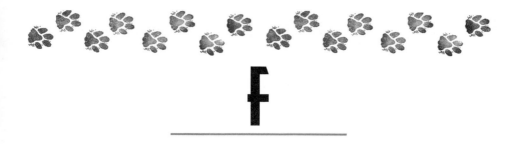

F

FATIGUE

Energize Your Dog with Apple-Cider Vinegar

Many years ago a country doctor by the name of D. C. Jarvis, M.D., who practiced in rural Vermont for a very long time, wrote a colorful book entitled *Folk Medicine*. It became an instant hit with a lot of people, who could easily relate to the practical wisdom contained in its pages.

The good doctor used two simple food items to give animals ranging from horses to hunting dogs and humans more energy—a common seaweed, kelp, and apple-cider vinegar (different from pickling or white vinegar). He had a friend who loved to hunt and kept a number of dogs around for that purpose. The friend asked Dr. Jarvis if he had anything to give his hounds that would help them not to tire so easily while out hunting with him.

Jarvis put the dogs on a relatively simple nutrition program. When they were not hunting they were to receive one teaspoon of kelp and one tablespoon of apple-cider vinegar in their rations every day. And when they did go out hunting, these amounts were doubled.

After three years of careful monitoring, the results were astonishing. Those dogs receiving the kelp and apple-cider vinegar every day hardly ever tired and were good for up to ten hours of steady hunting. Other dogs without it were only good for about three hours before they became pooped. The kelp-and-vinegar dogs also pointed and retrieved every bird for several hunters shooting into the air at the same time. The other dogs became easily disoriented and showed shortness of breath.

The supplemented dogs also had greater appetites and ate well. On the other hand, those dogs lacking the seaweed and apple-cider vinegar in their diets showed evidence of weight loss while hunting and didn't eat as heartily afterwards.

Dr. Jarvis believed that the iodine in the kelp and the fermented properties of the vinegar stimulated the thyroid and adrenal glands in these hunting dogs, enabling them to outperform the others. He felt that if more people would take both items on a regular basis as well as give them to their small animals, they and their pets would be a lot healthier and have more energy.

Chlorophyll Makes Super Pets out of Ordinary Dogs and Cats

For many years I've been a big fan of wheat and barley grasses grown in the soils of Lawrence, Kansas, where conditions are ideal for growing terrific chlorophyll. A dog food consisting of both cereal grasses, alfalfa, essential fatty acids (that include both omega 3 and 6), and several other things will give canines more energy than their owners ever imagined was possible. Cats benefit from this combination as well. (See Product Appendix under Pines for more information.)

I would also recommend adding a little liquid aged-garlic extract from Japan to these ingredients. (See Product Appendix under Wakunaga.) Bear in mind, though, that very active animals benefit from *some* organic meat, cats needing more of it than dogs do. Elsewhere in the book, as here, I advise a semi-vegetarian diet for pets instead of a complete one, since I believe that this is a much safer nutritional approach.

Super-Charged Meals for Pooped-Out Pets

Dr. Robert S. Goldstein and his wife, Susan, are nationally renowned experts in animal medicine and nutrition and animal emotional well-being. They are acquainted with my work and have several of my recently published health encyclopedias.

The Goldsteins edit a monthly international newsletter called *Love of Animals* that is devoted exclusively to the natural care and healing of people's pets. In their 1995 introductory issue they gave some food tips and meal suggestions for recharging the energy batteries in pooped-out pets. Here is what they wrote; it is used with their kind permission.

They begin the discussion by declaring in bold, black type: "Let's lift the ban on table scraps! It's fun and good for your animal." Then they mentioned what that morning's dog menu consisted of: "My leftover oatmeal, last night's organic baked potatoes with the skins, low-fat yogurt and organic carrots" added to a base of an organic brand of dog food they like. They state that table scraps like these have more vitality and nutritional goodness than do commercial pet foods.

"Sprinkling grated or chopped raw vegetables—particularly carrots—on the base food is the most important addition you can make if you want to do something very easy. Treat table scraps or leftovers as a supplement to your animal's daily diet. You will want to increase gradually the amount of living food and 'people' food you feed (especially if your animal has been dependent upon pet food).

"In our household, I make sure there are leftovers from each meal. If I'm making oatmeal, I make extra to share with my animals. . . . Collect raw vegetables from your salad (oil-free please, unless you are using extra-virgin oil alone) and any of the throwaway parts of vegetables (no moldy ones, of course) and leftover steamed veggies. Chop or grate and store in the refrigerator. There you have it! A healthy concoction at your fingertips.

"I like to keep my raw vegetables separate from the steamed. Raw foods will spoil faster because of the naturally occurring enzymes and bacteria. Try to use veggies within four to five days of preparation.

"Some of our [pets'] favorite veggies are carrots, Brussels sprouts, string beans, watercress and broccoli. Cats also love zucchini, cooked or raw. One vegetable to avoid . . . is the tomato.

"Our animals adore baked potatoes. If you don't have organic potatoes, scrub the skins well. Oats are great, as are all kinds of whole grains, such as brown rice and millet. Animals need roughage and fiber, just like you do. (Cat lovers: You'll have fewer hairballs to deal with when you increase the fiber.) Avoid foods made from refined wheat flour and white rice. . . .

"Fruits are good to serve with grains or as a snack. Organic apples and bananas are a favorite with our canines. They line up whenever I prepare fruit for [them]. Cats like melon. I never feed citrus to dogs or cats because it is too acidic.

"I don't serve my animals extra protein every meal or even every day. I play it by ear. But when I do serve it, I make sure it's quality meat, without residual hormones and pesticides. Good protein choices include: lean beef, and skinless, boneless chicken and fish (pick bones carefully). Tofu also is great (they will love it). If you can't buy organic meat, then leave off the skin since that's where the chemical residues are the highest. For meats, save out an unseasoned portion, cook slightly and serve. Avoid any meats or cuts that are prepared and chemically preserved, salted or sugared.

"To super-charge your animal's meals, here's what [we] recommend:

> *Chopped organic garlic:* Garlic is a . . . natural antibiotic . . . Chop up skins and all.
>
> *Extra-virgin olive oil:* . . . Olive oil . . . is highly digestible and will meet your dog's or cat's requirements for fat . . .
>
> *Low-fat organic plain yogurt:* Yogurt is [a] great source of predigested protein and fat.

"[Our] food plan is laid back in comparison to the rigid feeding instructions on pet food bags. The living foods, leftovers and extras are supplements to the amount of base food you're currently feeding. If you are adding a lot of extras one night, cut back on the base food. It's also important to tune into your animal's unique metabolism and to monitor his or her weight. Some breeds have a much slower metabolism than others.

"Just to give you an idea on proportions, here's what [we] would serve a 70 lb. dog and 10 lb. cat. These menus should give you the feel of the proportions so you can make your own judgment.

BREAKFAST

CANINE (70 LBS.)

1 ½ cups cooked oatmeal
2 tablespoons low-fat or nonfat plain yogurt
2 small baked potatoes (with skins present)
1 grated carrot
2 cups dry dog food

FELINE (10 LBS.)

¼ cup oatmeal
1 teaspoon low-fat yogurt
½ baked potato
¼ grated carrot
½ cup dry cat food

DINNER

CANINE (70 LBS.)

2 ½ cups dry dog food
1 tablespoon virgin olive oil
1 clove chopped garlic
2 stalks broccoli, chopped
¼ grated carrot

FELINE (10 LBS.)

¼ cup dry cat food
1 teaspoon virgin olive oil
½ clove chopped garlic
¼ small zucchini, chopped*
¼ chopped carrot*

*You will have to be determined, almost sneaky, when introducing veggies to cats. Start with ⅛ teaspoon chopped well and mix with moistened base food. Gradually increase."

FELINE LEUKEMIA

Some Interesting Facts

No less an authority than Richard H. Pitcairn, DVM had some interesting things to say about feline leukemia virus (FeLV), a retrovirus belonging to the same class that causes human AIDS. In *Dr. Pitcairn's Complete Guide to Natural Health for Dogs & Cats* (Emmaus, PA: Rodale Press, 1995; p. 272), the author made these several points concerning the disease:

- Approximately one quarter of all sick cats seen by veterinarians have FeLV.
- Cats between the ages of one to five years seem to be at highest risk.
- FeLV "occurs more often in neutered animals" than in unneutered males and females, though "no one knows why."
- Almost three-quarters of all cats are exposed to FeLV at some point in their lives, but recover on their own.
- Though there are several types of FeLV, they share the common symptoms of weight loss, fever, and dehydration.
- Cats that have had FeLV fail to reproduce properly. They're subject to automatic abortions, stillbirths, and giving births to weak kittens that fail to thrive in spite of excellent care given them.
- Fully one third of all cat tumors are a direct result of previous infection with FeLV.

Recognized Stages of Infection

Veterinarians know that there are basically six steps through which the feline leukemia virus progresses. Following is a summary of each:

FIRST STEP. Tissues of the oral cavity become infected; however, in healthy cats, the disease goes no further.

SECOND STEP. FeLV travels from the mouth to other parts of the cat's body via specific blood cells.

THIRD STEP. A cat's lymphatic system becomes infected. But even at this stage, a reasonably healthy cat can resist the disease from spreading further.

FOURTH STEP. Bone marrow becomes infected. When this happens, it's fairly certain that a cat will carry the disease for life, though proper treatment may help to control it.

FIFTH STEP. FeLV reinfects the blood through circulating cells.

SIXTH STEP. Various glands and organs are prone to continual infection: tear and salivary glands and the urinary bladder. An infected cat is now eliminating most of the virus and poses a danger to other healthy cats.

Ways of Coping with It

Veterinarians who practice alternative forms of healing (at least those I interviewed) acknowledge that diet invariably is to blame for a lot of the problems that pets incur. If continually fed a steady diet of commercial canned or packaged foods for long, animals will begin showing signs of physical infirmities. Such food, however delicious they may find it, isn't very nutritious. Even with the addition of synthetic vitamins, they don't provide well-balanced nutrition.

Animals, like humans, require a frequent diet of *raw* food teeming with life and vitality. Cooked food doesn't give this. The animal body (as its human counterpart) requires natural vitamins, strengthening minerals, activating enzymes, power-building amino acids, and stimulating fiber to give energy and stamina. It is virtually impossible to promote vigorous activity in any biological system for long without the benefit of wholesome, *un*cooked food.

The ideal, of course, would be for an animal or its human master to subsist entirely on organic, raw food. That type of steady diet would be of definite positive influence on health. There could almost be an unwritten guarantee that no sickness would ever visit such an animal or its master, at least not for long. But this way is neither practical nor affordable in the times we live. Some cooked food must of necessity be consumed now and then. The real trick comes in knowing how to find a balance between the two. The fine art of blending prepared food with raw and fresh doesn't take a college education to figure out. Just a little common sense, some careful shopping, and varying the mean intakes so that half is uncooked and the remainder prepared is about all that is required to enjoy reasonably good health.

This "50/50 diet" (as I've called it) pertains to animals as well as to humans. Your cat can be given canned items or your dog fed packaged food, but not every day. Raw vegetables, including uncooked meat, should be worked into their diets as well. This should be alternated with good food that is lightly cooked (preferably steamed, boiled, or baked). After this would come commercially prepared, store-bought foods.

Feline leukemia, just as nearly every other disease that affects innocent pets, is the end result of crummy feeding practices. Don't blame the cat or dog in such circumstances. Guilt rests squarely on the shoulders of pet owners, who carry their own careless buying and eating habits over to their domestic animals. Bad food lacking in good nutrition automatically weakens an animal's immune system. And when such defenses are down, viruses such as the one that causes feline leukemia creep in and take charge.

One of the first things that must be done in such cases is that the owner must adopt a course of stubborn determination, for his or her pet's life may hang in the balance. Diseases such as FeLV take away an animal's appetite, making recovery all the more difficult. No one likes to use force and nothing likes force exerted upon it. But sometimes in life-threatening situations, niceness must be laid aside and a certain amount of force must be used. An owner should understand that an infected cat will usually refuse to eat. Here the owner must make a tough decision, lay personal feeling aside, and *force-feed,* if necessary, a sick animal. Liquid food can be put down a cat's throat with a feeding syringe, although the task is both difficult and unpleasant.

I recommend the following food paste in such dire circumstances. It is extremely nutritious, tastes great, and above all is life-saving for a cat slowly dying of FeLV.

Life-Saving Food Paste

½ cup raw, organic beef liver

1 teaspoon Pines Mighty Greens*

1 teaspoon liquid Kyolic aged-garlic extract*

5 drops ConcenTrace*

1 teaspoon liquid vitamin C

or

1 tablet (260 mg.) vitamin C crushed to powder

4 tablespoons to ½ cup spring or mineral water as needed

*Consult the Product Appendix under Pines, Wakunaga, and Trace Minerals respectively for more information.

Put the ingredients in the order given into a Vita-Mix 5000 container. The amount of water to be used will be determined by the type of consistency desired. Less water will result in a paste, while nearly the full amount recommended will obviously yield a more liquefied solution. Secure the lid and run the machine for one-and-a-half minutes.

The paste can be scooped out with a flat wooden tongue depressor or a blunt-edged butter knife and scraped onto a cat's tongue once its mouth has been gently forced apart with a thickly gloved hand. Or the liquid can be put into a feeding syringe and inserted into the animal's mouth and given that way. Either operation takes time and requires considerable patience. Generally two people are required for this procedure, one to hold the animal's front paws down so it doesn't scratch and force its mouth open and the other to do the actual feeding.

It has been said by dedicated cat owners (and I firmly believe this) that if a loving, supportive attitude is constantly maintained toward a sick animal, it will respond better to treatments, even some of those it may not at first like. The suggestion of force is necessary only when all else fails and the animal utterly refuses to eat anything set before it.

The immune system of a sick cat responds well to raw protein food. Besides organic liver, there are also organic chicken, turkey, or lamb to consider. Raw organic eggs and cooked egg white or even tofu are other options to consider. Certain grains are wholesome, too. Cooked oatmeal, wheat, amaranth, quinoa (from South America), or wild rice will do a sick animal much good. Raw vegetables that can be grated, pureed, or juiced add valuable mineral salts to a sick animal's depleted system. Some of them can even be steamed or lightly cooked, if necessary. Favorites would include carrots, celery, string beans, Pontiac potatoes (the small red kind), and zucchini squash (when in season). But don't limit your pet just to these; expand your imagination to add asparagus, broccoli, corn (preferably canned), peas, sprouts (alfalfa, mung bean), or squash. Some of these would be better lightly boiled and then mashed or else juiced or pureed in their raw forms before feeding to a sick cat.

Of the many herb teas to consider for a problem such as this, I suggest red-clover blossoms. I've worked with this herb for many years in severe infections, including cancer. It is by far, I think, the best herb for detoxifying the body of poisons. To make a tea a sick cat will tolerate, add 2 teaspoons of red-clover blossoms and 1 teaspoon of dried catnip herb to 1½ pints boiling water (not tap). Cover, set aside, and steep for 20 minutes, or until cool. Strain and give kitty one-half cup in its water dish and refrigerate the rest. Reheat small amounts thereafter to room temperature before refilling its dish. Do not serve the tea cold.

Animal and Human Treatments Considered Together

This section is perhaps as good as anyplace to make a few interesting observations with regard to the treatment of sick pets. The many useful suggestions made in these pages are obviously intended for animals, as the title of the book implies. But just because they may be for someone's ailing cat or dog is no indication that they won't work for people too.

Some diseases are specific to the animal kingdom. The feline leukemia virus is one of these. And yet cannot a similar retrovirus (from the same oncovirus subfamily) that produces immunodeficiency and neoplastic disease be found in humans? We certainly have this among us in the form of AIDS.

Therefore, when treatment for animals is considered here, certain overlapping recommendations may be detected for human application as well. Take the use of aged-garlic extract, plant chlorophyll, vitamins and minerals, organic vegetables, wholesome grains, and red clover. All may be effectively incorporated into animal and human diets with good results. It is doubtful, though, that someone suffering from AIDS could relish, much less choke down, liver paste or catnip tea, which a cat infected with FeLV would most likely find quite palatable.

But there are enough dietary and supplemental parallels to suggest that what is good to give sick animals could very well benefit ailing people. Thus, the old adage that "What's good for the goose is good for the gander," may be restated as, "what's good for pets may be good for pet owners" when it comes to many remedial treatments. (Also see under Anorexia for additional data.)

FEVERS

The Good, Bad, and Ugly

Fevers occur in animals and humans as a consequence of bacterial or viral infections. But they do have their good side, believe it or not. Andre Lwoff was the first to question the idea that fever was an intrinsic part of the disease process and thus a phenomenon to be vigorously combated with drugs. This somewhat eccentric Nobel laureate was working at the Pasteur Institute in Paris in the late 1960s when he discovered that the poliomyelitis virus grew well in tissue-cultured cells at 95° F. but did poorly as the temperature approached 104° F. He and his colleagues found that when dogs infected with the polio-virus vaccine were given fever-reducing drugs, their chances of dying dramatically increased. But when left alone and given only adequate water and plenty of time to rest, they improved remarkably.

The bad side to fevers, of course, is that they can make us and our pets very uncomfortable. Physical systems automatically become weakened as body temperatures rise:

Normal temperature in a human is 98.6° F.

Normal temperature in a cat is about 100.2° F.

Normal temperature in a dog is about 102.8° F.

Obviously anything over these respective figures constitutes a feverish state.

Fevers become ugly when they're prolonged (between 105° and 106° F.) and can lead to dehydration, anorexia, mental and emotional depression, cerebral edema, bone-marrow depression, and hallucinations. If left unchecked at these temperatures, they could turn fatal.

Fever Busters

During their initial phase, fevers seldom are a serious problem so long as they don't escalate into the stratosphere too quickly. The medical evidence shows that fevers are in themselves an important defense mechanism. The bodies of humans and animals are much wiser than we are. We should not attempt to interfere with normal physiological responses to illness just because we have the drug arsenal to do so.

There are several wonderful herbs that make outstanding "fever busters" (as I term them). These plants are of the mint family and should be taken in liquid (tea, fluid extract, tincture) rather than capsule or tablet forms. They belong to the mint family and taste great: catnip (which felines go crazy over), spearmint (which drives some dogs ecstatic, strange to say), and peppermint (which their human masters seem to like a lot).

To one-and-a-half pints of boiling spring or distilled water, add one heaping tablespoon of any one of these three herbs. Cover, set aside, and steep for 30 minutes. Strain and have the animal drink this instead of water.

Fever Miracle

One herb that always seems to perform a "Mike Tyson knockout" in the fever ring is wormwood. It is bitter as gall, therefore, getting it down the gullet as a tea is a tall order, indeed. Instead use only one capsule for small pets (cats) and no more than two capsules for bigger ones (dogs).

The Chinese have been using wormwood for several thousand years and consider it to be a "fever miracle" for rapidly eradicating the symptoms common to this problem.

Fleas

The Average Flea

A flea is a small (under one-half inch), wingless insect of the order *Siphonaptera,* of which there are approximately 1,600 species. The average flea has a laterally flattened body with bristles and spines known as ctenidia. The flea's mouthparts are especially adapted for piercing and sucking, hence the name of *Siphon*aptera. A flea's legs are so developed as to allow for incredible leaping. One very athletically inclined flea broke a record with a 4-foot vertical high jump. (If a man had equal ability, one leap would cover five city blocks.)

The black specks found on household pets and in their sleeping areas are really nothing more than "flea calling cards." Such paper-like particles are actually dried blood, commonly called flea dirt. They are an essential part of the average flea's life cycle. Understanding this cycle will enable you to get the upper hand in terms of controlling fleas around your pets.

An adult female flea ingests blood (up to 15 times its own bodyweight) and commences laying eggs. These eggs drop off the host animal into the surrounding environment and hatch into larvae in a very short time (2 to 12 days as a rule). The larvae feed on dried blood, flea feces, and other debris, going through three stages of development in eight days to three weeks. The larvae live wherever the eggs have fallen and develop into the cocoon stage. The presence of cats, dogs, and their human owners stimulate the cocoon to emerge as a young adult flea.

This adult flea has been uniquely adapted for a parasitic existence in body size and structure. It feeds exclusively on the blood of mammals and birds. One flea usually eats twice a day, but has the capacity to exist a couple of months before feeding again. Also, a flea usually lives up to eight months once it begins sucking blood.

Fleas multiply faster than rabbits or frogs. Just one female flea is capable of laying 50 eggs per day for a potential total of 160,000 offspring in about two months. What this tells us is that if you find one flea on your cat or dog, chances are good that an entire community of them are hiding out in the animal's fur and bedding and even in your carpet. Therefore, in order to effectively rid your pet of fleas, you must also treat your home and yard at the same time, otherwise you'll be fighting a losing battle.

Take Them Seriously

Many pet owners dismiss fleas as a mere annoyance for themselves and their pets. But this is a B-I-G mistake. Since most fleas change hosts quite often, they become significant disease carriers. Fleas are known to cause anemia, flea allergies, flea-bite dermatitis, occasional fever, periodic fatigue, and tapeworms.

In rare cases, they can pass bubonic plague from an infected host to you or your pet. In 1995, the Centers for Disease Control reported seven cases of bubonic plague, including one fatality, in Arizona, California, New Mexico, and Oregon. The majority of these occurred on the Navajo Indian reservation and came from dogs owned by individual tribal members.

An old nursery rhyme that many of our parents or grandparents taught us as children, begins, "Ring around the rosies, a pocket full of posies . . ." It might be of some historical interest to you to know that this specifically refers to the effect of bubonic plague spread by flea bites in Europe and Asia in the fourteenth century. "Ring around the rosies" refers to the red rashes that developed around flea bites. And "a pocket full of posies" refers to nosegays, the small bunches of flowers that people in those times always carried in hopes of perfuming the air around them, with the idea of countering the smell of death.

Two Types of Fleas

If you're one of the estimated 137 million Americans who owns a cat or dog, you'll probably want to know a little about the two basic kinds of fleas that afflict such creatures. There is also another one that is more common to humans, but can cross over to dogs, hogs, and even poultry if it desires.

The cat flea *(Ctenocephalides felis)* is roughly .08 of an inch in length and has worldwide distribution. The male is always a tad shorter than the female. Although generally found on cats, this species also parasitizes dogs, humans, other mammals, and poultry.

With the aid of a powerful magnifying glass or microscope, it can be easily distinguished from the dog flea by its sloping forehead.

The dog flea *(Ctenocephalides canis)* coexists with canines all over the globe. The male is about .08 of an inch long, with the female being slightly larger—.14 of an inch long. This species is distinguished from the cat flea by a round forehead. Besides dogs, it also feeds on the blood of cats and humans.

Finally, there is the human flea *(Pulex irritans),* which is reddish brown in color and between 0.8 and .12 of an inch long. It also has worldwide distribution. The life span ranges from several months to one-and-a-half years. This species can live for one-half year or more without eating. But it does require blood before mating. Its bite becomes painful after several days.

Leeuwenhoek's Fleas

One of the greatest scientists of the seventeenth century was a Dutchman named Antonie van Leeuwenhoek. He was the first person ever to observe bacteria, protozoa, and fleas through a lens. His accurate interpretations of what he saw eventually led to the sciences of bacteriology and protozoology a century later.

As a young man he established himself as a draper and haberdasher. By obtaining a coveted position as chamberlain to the sheriffs of Delft, Holland, he secured for himself an annual income that was sufficiently large to enable him to devote much of his private time to his all-absorbing hobby of grinding lenses.

Leeuwenhoek's methods of microscopy, which he kept secret, remain something of a mystery today. He ground over 400 lenses during his lifetime, most of which were very small—some no larger than a pinhead—and usually mounted them between two thin brass plates, riveted together. A large sample of these lenses, bequeathed to the Royal Society of England, were found to have magnifying powers of between 50 and, at the most, 300 times. In order to observe phenomena as infinitely tiny as bacteria, Leeuwenhoek must have employed some form of oblique illumination, or other technique, for enhancing the effectiveness of the lens, but this method he would not reveal.

In 1674 he began to observe bacteria and protozoa, which he isolated from a number of different sources as varying as pond water and saliva secretions from the human mouth. In 1677 he described for the first time the spermatozoa from insects, dogs, and human. In 1680, he noticed that yeasts consist of minute globular particles. In 1684 he gave the first accurate description of red blood cells.

A friend put him in touch with the Royal Society, to which he communicated by means of informal letters most of his discoveries from 1673 until August 26, 1723, when he quietly passed away at home at the age of 90 (something incredible in those times of much shorter life spans). He was elected a fellow to this prestigious scientific society in 1680. His discoveries were for the most part made public in the Society's *Philosophical Transactions*. In fact, the first representation ever made of bacteria is to be found in a hand sketch drawn by himself for that publication in 1683.

His letter on the flea is, perhaps, one of the most intriguing of all, so far as scientific discoveries for that century went. The common assertion by many then was that the flea originated from sand or dust. But Leeuwenhoek took some samples of live fleas from his Yorkshire terrier, put them on white foolscap paper, and then employed his curious method of microscopy to observe them. In his letter to the Society, he not only described a flea's physical structure but likewise traced out the entire history of its metamorphosis. The exactness of his observations enabled people, for the first time, to understand something about "this minute and despised creature," which Leeuwenhoek opposed on account of its "spontaneous generation" (or ability to reproduce itself so rapidly).

He demonstrated that this tiny creature was "endowed with as great perfection in its kind as any large animal" and proved that it bred in the regular way of winged insects. Besides fleas, he also carefully studied ants, sea mussel, and eels, which were at that time presumed to originate from dew. But it was his work on fleas, bacteria, and protozoa, above anything else, that made him world renowned and earned the respect of many notables, including the Queen of England and Peter the Great of Russia.

Leeuwenhoek's Methods of Preventing Flea Infestation

The Dutchman made 375 contributions to the *Philosophical Transactions* of the Royal Society of England and slightly over two dozen to the *Memoirs of the Paris Academy of Sciences*. Two collections of his works appeared during his life, one in Dutch (1685–1718) and the other in Latin (1715–1722). A selection was translated by S. Hoole and published under the title of *The Select Works of A. van Leeuwenhoek* (1798–1807). Unfortunately, Hoole's work omitted much of the material with regard to flea control. I had to go back to the primary sources in order to obtain the information given here in this section (some with the help of interpreters who understood Dutch and Latin).

In Leeuwenhoek's time it was popular for men to wear wigs. A portrait done of him by the famous Dutch master Jan Verkolje that now hangs in Amsterdam's Rijksmuseum shows the man sitting beside a small table wearing a long silk coat and a shoulder-length wig. In those days wigs were a distinctive class symbol, covering the back and shoulders. Women also wore them sometimes, but less often than the men did.

The wig would be removed at night and carefully set aside before the individual retired to bed. Left unattended this way, the average wig became an ideal nesting place for fleas. Many wig wearers, therefore, were continually bothered with the biting and itching these nasty, little creatures inflicted upon them. Leeuwenhoek mentioned being bothered by them and what course he took to rid himself of them. "I started eating a clove [of raw garlic] a day. It had the good effect of driving these miserable and minute creatures away from me. I suspect that the odors of this smelly herb were the chief reason they vacated my head covering."

Believing that his beloved Yorkshire terrier might be the cause and carrier of them, he carefully inspected the dog's coat and confirmed his suspicions. He devised an effective herbal powder with which he dusted his pet three or four times a week. Leeuwenhoek's herbal flea powder consisted of equal parts of the following dried and crushed herbs: eucalyptus, fennel, fleabane, garlic, onion, rosemary, rue, tansy, and wormwood. He kept this herbal mixture stored in a glass jar and away from sunlight.

He did a "backwards combing" by running his fingers through the animal's coat in the opposite direction from which it grew. With each raking he would introduce a little powder into the base of the hairs. He gave more attention to the little terrier's neck, back, and stomach than anywhere else, believing that in those places fleas congregated the most. The result after a number of weeks doing this is that "my dog no longer scratches himself and is completely free of these atrocious creatures."

Other Remedies

Besides the herbs that Leeuwenhoek utilized for flea control, there are a few other things that work nearly as well. One of these is the use of pyrethrum products made from the dried and crushed flowers of chrysanthemums. They are quite effective and can be safely used indoors without harming pets or crawling infants. Such powders should be applied on floors, along baseboards, beneath pet sleeping areas, and anywhere else you can think of that insects may try to hide.

Several essential oils can be especially helpful, but *never* apply them directly to an animal's skin as they will cause a great deal of irritation and discomfort. Instead, add a few drops of tea tree, eucalyptus, or pennyroyal oil to a bottle of natural shampoo (I prefer Mane & Tail) or a good-quality castile soap. Bathing your cat or dog with either of these is a safe, effective way to kill fleas. Dogs can be bathed once a week. But as you know just how much cats hate water, you should shampoo them only once a month or every six weeks at the most.

An herbal tea made from sour citrus fruits is of value in getting rid of fleas on your pet. Thinly slice an *un*peeled lemon and lime. Pour one pint of boiling water over them, cover with a lid, and let them steep overnight. Strain and put into an empty sprayer bottle and spray onto the animal's coat and leave it to dry. Or you can sponge it on your pet's skin for a more thorough saturation.

I recommend adding 15 drops of fennel, garlic, lavender, pennyroyal, rosemary, sage, or sandalwood liquid extract to the preceding mixture prior to spraying it on the animal. One or even several of these herbs will boost the anti-flea properties of this citrus spray, making it even more potent. (Consult the Product Appendix under Nature's Answer to obtain any of these herbs.)

Basic Flea Prevention

Prevention is always the easiest way to keep something unpleasant from occurring. It requires constant diligence, a great deal of effort, and a lot of time. Since fewer steps are involved in preventing a major flea infestation, it also means less money spent on flea-control products, not to mention avoiding all the hassle involved in ridding your home and pet of fleas.

Vacuum every inch of floor space several times a week. This includes shag carpeting and bare hardwood floors. Get even areas your cat or dog doesn't go on, such as under the sofa. Be sure to dispose of the vacuum bags in an outside trash bin that will soon be emptied. If you don't do this or if you place the bag in an inside garbage bin, the fleas are bound to escape, and your cleaning efforts will have been in vain. Clean any surface where a flea could hide, which basically means everywhere. Don't forget the easy chair, the ottoman, or the end tables. Here's a handy hint: Place a flea collar or segment of one inside your vacuum bag (if it isn't the disposable kind) to kill adult fleas that might escape. Also, if using a disposable bag, discard it immediately after vacuuming even if it isn't completely full. Otherwise, your vacuum bag could become a "food-filled" harbor for developing eggs and larvae.

It is a good idea to use a flea-control spray outdoors. If left untreated, your yard could harbor a flea population that can work its way back into even the most meticulously cleaned house. Spray your dog's entire habitat, concentrating on shady areas and areas it frequents the most. And if you have ants outside, leave them alone. Ants love dining on flea eggs and larvae, which is a good enough reason to forego pesticides that kill all yard insects.

Be sure to mow and water your lawn regularly. Short grass permits the sunlight to heat up the soil. This kills any flea larvae that may be secreted in it. And watering helps to drown any fleas in the developing stages of life. You can sterilize bare earth believed to contain fleas by covering it with heavy black-plastic sheeting. The buildup of heat beneath the plastic does a great job of killing fleas and their larvae.

Finally, get some agricultural lime (*not* the kind used in construction work) and pour a little cayenne pepper in with it (one cup of cayenne for every one gallon of lime). Mix well with a stick and then spread evenly on grassy or moist areas to help dry out the fleas. For additional flea control in your yard think about using nematodes; these are microscopic worms that prey on insect larvae and pupae. When the fleas disappear, so will the worms. Look for them at pet and garden stores and follow label directions for usage.

Natural, unrefined diatomaceous earth is highly recommended for combating fleas in your yard, but it isn't to be used inside. Comprised of fossilized shell remains of single-celled algae, diatomaceous earth is finely ground and resembles a sort of chalky dust. It effectively kills fleas by destroying the waxy coating that covers their external skeletons. But direct contact with the material is harmless to cats and dogs and humans. Care should be taken, however, to avoid breathing it into the lungs.

Keep food in sealed containers or in the refrigerator. Remove and clean your cat's or dog's dishes after it eats. Wipe up crumbs and spills, disposing of them in containers with tight-fitting lids. And wipe out standing water in sinks, tubs, and shower stalls.

Nutrition, the Frontline Defense

The last and most important step in basic flea prevention is making sure your household pet gets the kind of food that can stimulate its ability to resist parasites such as fleas. Look for those marketed as super-premium, natural pet foods formulated to provide 100 percent complete and balanced nutrition, but lacking chemical preservatives such as ethoxyquin, BHA or BHT, artificial flavors, or appetite stimulants.

I suggest working several types of supplementary items into your pet's daily food. Adding a little powdered brewer's yeast, liquid Kyolic garlic, a few drops of liquid mineral ConcenTrace, a sprinkle of crushed tablets of zinc powder, and some barley grass concentrate to *moist* food will strengthen an animal's immune defenses against illnesses brought on by fleas. And as they get worked into the system, a peculiar but not necessarily unpleasant hint of body odor is emitted that fleas intensely dislike but is scarcely discernible to human detection. (Consult the Product Appendix under Naturally Vitamins, Wakunaga, Trace Minerals, and Pines for further information on the previously mentioned supplements.)

A Place Where Fleas Flourish

I can think of nothing better to close this section with than reciting for readers a place where fleas actually flourish because certain humans want them to. I'm speaking, of course, about the research-and-development facility appropriately called Flea World. It is operated by the Heska Corporation of Fort Collins, Colorado. Heska is a major manufacturer of the Heska Flea Allergy Dermatitis (FAD) Test and usually raises about 300,000 fleas weekly.

It is believed to be the largest flea-breeding facility anywhere in North America. A team of 5 full-time and 12 part-time employees keeps Flea World open 365 days a year. Currently Heska is developing the first dog and cat flea-control vaccine, expected to provide extended protection against fleas. The company launched initial testing at the beginning of 1997 to detect whether a dog is allergic to flea bites and not to the flea body or other insects. Their FAD measures a dog's immune reaction to portions of flea saliva, which is injected when the flea bites and causes a flea-allergic dog's skin to redden and itch.

It's difficult for fleas to escape, since the entire facility's tile floors, ceilings, walls, and countertops are all white. And researchers wear white laboratory coats to make detection of a fugitive flea easier.

Actress June Lockhart's Herbal Secret for Flea Management in Pets

Those of us old enough to know would recognize the name of June Lockhart, the well-known star of the long-running television series *Lassie,* which many of us grew up with as kids. For the last few years she has been starring in a new role as a celebrity spokesperson for an organization that places trained dogs with the deaf. She is an enthusiastic supporter for International Hearing Dog, Inc., of Henderson, Colorado.

In the last decade this small organization has trained and placed more than 500 dogs in homes in the United States and Canada. All the canines come from animal shelters and would have been put to sleep if a home hadn't been found for them. They are usually sensitive, smaller, mixed-breed dogs.

"It's quite a wonderful program," Ms. Lockhart told a newspaper reporter not long ago. "Everyone wins. The deaf have a companion, and the dogs are not put to sleep. And they usually get to live in wonderful places besides!"

The dogs are selected for intelligence, adaptability, and eagerness to please and are trained for about three months before they are given free to a deaf person. They are trained to respond to important household sounds: a crying baby, smoke alarm, telephone, alarm clock, a doorbell, a security buzzer, or to danger. "They are now training dogs for people who are both deaf *and* blind," Ms. Lockhart noted. "This is a very difficult task. It can be quite tricky and requires a lot of patience on the part of the trainer."

One of the problems that has faced deaf owners of such specially trained dogs in the past has been that of fleas. But Ms. Lockhart discovered for herself, quite by accident, the virtues of liquid Kyolic garlic, which is a potent extract of aged garlic from Japan. "I bought a few bottles myself of this Kyolic for my own dogs and the flea problem ended almost immediately," she informed the journalist. She sprinkled some of the liquid on their chow every day for prompt flea control.

She passed this tip along to the folks at the International Hearing Dog, Inc. In turn, the idea was suggested in writing to new candidates for their dogs, with good results. It is recommended that Kyolic Super Formula 101 (two tablets) or one-half teaspoon of Kyolic Liquid be used three times a day for a week with cats and toy dog breeds, and two tablets or one-half teaspoon once a day thereafter for maintenance of general health. For medium-sized dogs and cats, the dosage should be increased to four tablets of one teaspoon three times daily for one week, and four tablets or one teaspoon a day thereafter for health-maintenance purposes. For large dogs, Ms. Lockhart believes that eight tablets or one tablespoon, three times a day for one week, will help to remove even the most stubborn intestinal parasites and fleas. Thereafter, six or eight tablets or one tablespoon daily of the liquid aged-garlic extract should be given to maintain optimal health in bigger canines. (Consult the Product Appendix under Wakunaga of America for more information.)

(Also see Skin Problems for additional data.)

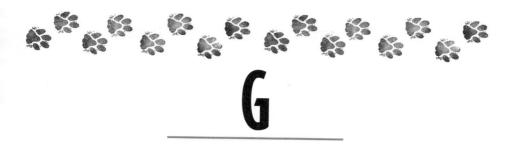

G

GROOMING

Well-Groomed Beagles Sniff out Trouble

These days many of the comic strips featured in the comics section of most daily newspapers are nothing much to laugh about. But occasionally a comic strip comes along that reflects a genuine sense of humor in the illustrator. Such a one is *Fred Basset* drawn by A. Graham and distributed by the Chicago Tribune Media Services. Being British obviously helps, for the cartoonist invests some of that dry wit (for which his people are famous) into every featured drawing.

I am reminded of one strip in particular that appeared in the Tuesday, February 3, 1998, Section C of the *Salt Lake Tribune*. Fred, the lovable and friendly basset hound, is leashed outside a store near a parking meter. An old woman approaches and remarks, "Aha, a beagle! Beagles are my favorite dog, you know." Whereupon Fred looks at her inquisitively while she bends forward to pat his head and thinks to himself: "'Beagle'? With all due respect, madam, I think you need new glasses!"

Well, the genuine article (that is *real* beagles) are used in a number of Western states for a variety of smelling jobs: Six of them were dispatched from California to an exploded chemical factory outside Reno, Nevada, in January 1998 to search for victims; another beagle named Annie greeted passengers coming off international flights in San Francisco, alert for the scent of forbidden food; and in Hawaii, beagles belonging to a canine agricultural-inspection team checked packages for the odor of snake.

The noses of dogs have been known for many generations to be powerfully sensitive. Smell is their most acute sense—perhaps

500,000 times more potent than humans' abilities to detect odors. But beagles' sense of smell is almost double that, probably like a million times. Beagles are even thought to surpass bloodhounds, the ultimate canine sniffing machines.

Historically, dogs have been chiefly used for hunting game and tracking fugitives. But today canines of all species (other than beagles)—German shepherds, Labradors, Dobermans, and St. Bernards—are being employed in a widening range of jobs, some quite specialized. Their targets could be illegal drugs or bear gallbladders, smuggled explosives, or lost children. If an object has a scent, a dog can be trained to search for it, handlers declare.

I had one such dog-handling coordinator at San Francisco's International Airport (who wished to remain anonymous for security reasons) tell me: "In the age of high-tech electronics, man's best friend is still the best friend we have." "Why beagles in particular?" I asked. "Because they're more adorable and less threatening than, say, a police dog or mastiff. People who get caught with prohibited foods are less inclined to be irritated when caught by canines than by human agricultural inspectors. In fact, many of them think it's a 'fun thing' that our beagles found their stashed food."

I complimented my informant on several beagles he and a couple of assistants had with them at the time of our interview. "These are *very* nice-looking dogs," I stated. "We try hard to keep them looking good and in great shape" he replied.

Food Assimilation More Important than Diet

I mentioned to my informant that I'd read in a few alternative-care pet books about diet being the main thing in contributing toward a pet's external appearance. I was astonished when this individual said, "Quite frankly, we think it lies in good food *assimilation!*" Noticing my look of amazement, he continued: "We've tried some of the best organic foods on the market and have brushed our dogs till the sun set, but with only minimal results. It wasn't until we started giving them a product from Canada that a *big* difference was noticed!"

He then told me a little bit about what was called Bio-K+. "It comes from Montreal, I believe. It was developed by some famous

French guy, a Doctor _____." Not remembering the name, we went back to his office, where he shuffled through a pile of papers stuffed in one drawer until he found the sheet he was looking for. "Here, I'll let you read it," he said as he thrust the page into my hands.

The information sheet said that the scientist with the difficult-pronouncing name, Dr. François-Marie Luquet, a renowned micro-biologist who has been affiliated with France's well-known Pasteur Institute, created a unique blend of two acidophilus strains, *Lactobacillus acidophilus* and *Lactobacillus casei,* that are currently being marketed for the first time as a fermented milk product.

"We give each of our beagles half of one small container (3.5 oz.)," the canine coordinator said. "We just mix it in with their food. They really seem to take to the stuff. I've tried some of it myself, and it doesn't taste bad at all. But you gotta keep it refrigerated or else it goes flat and is no longer active. We started noticing a change right away, maybe in a week or less, with our dogs' coats, how much glossier they became. And—you might find this interesting—there was a lot *less* 'doggie breath' in each of them. We figure this 'Quebec yogurt,' as we jokingly call it around here, helps the beagles to assimilate their food much better and does away with those diges-tive after-odors you smell on a dog's breath so often."

I contacted the company in Montreal, which has exclusive North American distribution rights for Bio-K+. Claude Chevalier, for-merly head of the Dairy Bureau of Canada, mentioned that ongoing research is continuing to be done with leading medical organizations in Canada and elsewhere pertaining to the product's human health benefits: lowers serum cholesterol, especially "bad" or LDL choles-terol by as much as 35 percent, which helps to reduce the risk of heart attacks; stabilizes intestinal flora which promotes better diges-tion and assimilation; and boosts immune defenses.

Mr. Chevalier told me of one situation in which a Quebecois woman of 36, a schoolteacher named Cécile Chicoutimi, residing in Saint-Anne de la Pocatière, after having used the product herself to cor-rect a gastrointestinal problem, started applying a little bit to some of the hot spots on her dog's back with incredible results. "The sores disap-peared and the hair grew back within a couple of weeks," Claude said.

(See Product Appendix under Bio-K+ International for more information.)

Pomeranian Power Takes Blue Ribbons at Dog Shows

Stephanie Drysdale loves her Pomeranian pooches very much. She ought to because they're both g-r-e-a-t-looking dogs and have taken various Pomeranian dog shows by storm in the last few years. "I keep my animals *very* healthy!" she said matter-of-factly during a recent visit following the Natural Foods Expo East convention, where we met at one of my several book signings.

"The reason my animals' coats look simply divine," she said with an air of self-importance (and a touch of vanity, too, I might add), "is that I see to it they each get the proper balance of essential fatty acids and biotin (a B vitamin)." I could tell from the way she talked that this lady had done her homework when it came to animal nutrition. "The essential fatty acids make their coats thicker and shinier, while biotin works as a nutritional enzyme for their complete synthesis." She obtains these things from a local health-food store in the Baltimore area.

"I combine one-half teaspoon of the oils of flaxseed and sunflower together and then mix in one-quarter teaspoon powdered biotin with it. This I work into their food twice a day. The results have been most impressive." At her home a day later, she showed me a wall full of framed blue-ribbon prizes and certificates her two dogs had handily won in a number of shows around the country. "These supplements have also stopped excessive shedding, improved their doggy odors and drippy eyes, and eliminated both dry and oil skins, eczema, and hot spots."

The Cat that Built an Entire Pet-Products Company

Some 12 years ago, Andi Brown's Maine coon cat, a male named Spot, developed a diseased condition that conventional veterinary care and prescription drugs or premium commercial foods couldn't correct. "It manifested itself," she told me by telephone recently, "as skin and coat disorders and eye discharges. He had a horrendous odor that would clear out Palm Harbor [Florida] down here. I've never smelled anything so awful in my life!"

She met a friend who was into "the holistic bit." He visited her house and saw the sick animal and made inquiry into its diet. She showed him the expensive brand of dog food that her vet had recommended. He told her that "what I was feeding my pet was actually the cause of all its woes!" He showed her how to prepare a stew made with organic chicken parts, wild rice, and fresh vegetables.

I asked her what this stew contained. "Oh, heavens, you would have to ask something like that," she said in mild frustration. "Let's see . . . we made our first batch in a ten-quart stainless-steel pot. I believe a medium-sized chicken was used. Besides this we chopped up and included: one garlic bulb, four stalks of celery, four carrots, a handful of green beans, four zucchinis, four yellow squash, and a handful of green peas. Later on, when we expanded it for dogs, we added one cup of rolled oats, one cup of barley, and one cup of pasta (elbow macaroni)."

Within five days and ten feedings of this stew, "Spot turned into the most gorgeous and healthy cat you'd ever want to lay eyes upon. Even now as we're speaking, he's sitting right here in my lap purring away." As they began sharing her friend's recipe with a number of other pet owners and realizing the fantastic results they were getting, "the decision was made to go into business." The result of Spot's health turnaround with a wonderful homemade stew was a company called Purely for Pets.

And out of that same recipe grew her best-selling product, Dream Coat. She included the oils of garlic, evening primrose, wheat germ, safflower, sunflower, and soy. Cats get one-half teaspoon and bigger dogs two teaspoons per day in their food. The idea is to restore those essential fatty acids that have been processed out of most commercial pet foods. (See the Product Appendix under Purely for Pets for additional details.)

Three Supplements for Putting the Shine Back in Your Pet's Coat

Toni Dickerson of Westminster, Maryland, always uses the liquid version of Japanese aged-garlic extract in her dog's food to give him a nice coat. She has shared her simple success story with others. "I was walking my dog one day when I met an older woman with a feisty boxer. She was worrying about his health, particularly his skin, which was covered with hot spots and bumps. She'd tried medication, change of diet, everything the vet had suggested but with no luck.

"I recounted my own success with liquid garlic from Japan and encouraged her to add some of it to Buster's food. I didn't meet Buster again until several months later. When I did, his 'mom' became ecstatic. 'Look at Buster's skin!' she exclaimed. 'He's all better now, thanks to you.' Sure enough, Buster's golden-brown skin was silky smooth and blemish-free." Both women added one teaspoon of liquid Kyolic to their dogs' food twice daily. (See Product Appendix under Wakunaga.)

Mabel Winters is a resident of Portland, Maine. She gives her cat Cheshire (named after the mythical cat with the broad grin in Lewis Carroll's endearing children's novel *Alice's Adventures in Wonderland*) his allotment of silicon with his daily rations. "I crush one tablet and sprinkle it into his food once a day," she related. "His hair is so beautiful that he is the envy of the bridge club when it's my turn to host them. Some of them want to take him home and claim him for themselves, but I won't let them." (See Product Appendix under Scandinavian Naturals for more data.)

Finally, a great "skin success story" from my animal-lovers friends Dr. Robert and Susan Goldstein, editors of the monthly newsletter *Love of Animals* (see Appendix II for subscription information). Many of their health-care and nutritional ideas are located elsewhere in this book, as well as more details about them and how we met. So, with their permission, I'll cut right to the chase and quote the wonderful story they related in the march 1996 issue of their publication.

"Putting the shine back in [our dog] Jack's coat is one of many success stories [we've] had with ACV [apple-cider vinegar]. My favorite story involves a mangy old dog named Nick, who probably had never seen a veterinarian in his whole life. Nick's human companion stumbled on to [our] store [Lick Your Chops in Manhattan] a few years ago accompanied by his scroungy canine, who had horrible eczema, which had created large patches of bare, scaly skin. This poor little dog would have broken your heart! I wanted to recommend every product I knew of to help, but I started with simple, cheap apple-cider vinegar.

"We didn't see or hear from them for six months. Then, one day the man pulled up in his old pickup. To my astonishment, the little dog showed off a beautiful, full coat without a trace of eczema. The man proudly explained that Nick received ACV [apple-cider vinegar] religiously, every day.

"Nick no doubt needed a good dose of easily absorbed, natural minerals. . . . Even dogs like Jack who are on a good diet show off the extra minerals with a shinier coat [thanks to ACV]." Apple-cider vinegar is available at health food stores and supermarkets.

My Own Grooming Success Tips

Isn't it wonderful how different pet owners have discovered simple solutions to improving the skin and coat conditions of their animals? That's been one of the real pleasures in doing this book for my publisher. I'm able to bring together a lot of valuable information from many different sources for the benefit of people like yourself. Now let me share with you my own health tips for successful pet grooming.

There is a desert herb called yucca that grows in the American West and Southwest. It is a fantastic supplement to give *any* animals. Yucca is currently being used in some dog, cat, horse, cattle, and poultry feed for several reasons. For one thing, it reduces the noxious odor in urine and feces. In studies that examined the chemical breakdown of urea (the body's final by-product of digested proteins), it was discovered that the anhydrous ammonia, which is the main cause of the less than delightful smell of animal excrement, is produced by a single microbial enzyme called *urease*. Further studies indicated that food supplements of yucca tend to inhibit the production of urease, and as a result, fecal and urine odors are reduced by up to 56 percent in dogs and 49 percent in cats. People who feed yucca to reduce odors usually aren't aware of the nutritional role it plays in this equation. Poor-quality proteins produce excess urea and larger, more offensive stools. But with yucca frequently in their diets, animals and poultry are given more balance to their gastrointestinal tracts so that excess fecal and urine odor cease to be an issue.

The mystique surrounding yucca's impressive track record as a nutritional supplement and medicinal agent is probably due to its active ingredients. Sarspogenin and smilagenin, known to scientists as phytosterols or steroidal saponins, are precursors to the body's own naturally produced corticosteroids. These body substances prevent arthritis and psoriasis from occurring and are critical to the health of bone joints and skin.

But just because yucca is a tremendous herb doesn't mean an animal should receive it every day. My general recommendation is that a pet receive the emptied contents from two capsules of yucca (about one teaspoon) every *other* day and then *only* in just one meal. Adding a complete B vitamin of one-half teaspoon brewer's yeast with this works even better.

Finally, I prescribe Rex Wheat Germ Oil to all creatures, both great and small, two-legged as well as four-legged. Cats and small dogs get one-half teaspoon every day while larger dogs receive one tablespoon. (See Product Appendix under Anthropological Research Center to order.) Both of these items together make animal grooming a smashing success.

The Goldstein Program for Smart Grooming

I now return to my friends, Bob and Susan—the information they wanted me to share with my readers comes from two principal sources: a booklet, *The Goldstein Program for Healthy Animals,* and the January 1996 *Love of Animals* newsletter.

"A beautiful coat *is* skin deep," they insist. They suggest as a good New Year's or anytime resolution to make "beautiful fur a mission in your house" if you own a pet or two. It certainly is so in their abode. "But we don't start with the fur itself, we start with the skin. Beautiful fur is a reflection of healthy skin, and the skin absolutely reveals your animal's true state of health."

For want of space, I've capsulated their considerable information into the following short summary:

1. Brush and comb an animal's coat *all year round,* not just seasonally such as, say, in the spring. "Brush and comb your friend at least weekly." But "instead of the standard grooming brush," they recommend brushing the pet "with a dry loofah or body brush," which can be purchased from any pharmacy or health-food store. This type of skin stimulation "encourages the body's natural oils to surface and opens the pores. You can use the loofah dry or with water and shampoo. Massage your dog or cat using short, horizontal strokes starting at the head and neck and moving down the back to the belly and legs. This technique gently massages many key acupressure points, making this treatment much more than cosmetic. The body brush is a stiff brush with natural bristles sold in health-food stores or bath shops. It usually is sold with a long handle. The brush itself can be removed and fits comfortably in your hand with a strap for clutching. Use the brush the same way you would the loofah." Both of these instruments are also great skin workouts for pet *owners,* I might add.

2. Rejuvenate your animal with clean water. Dogs and cats are made up of two-thirds water, so water must be taken seriously. Water is a great rejuvenator. It flushes toxins from the body, contributes to the feeling of well-being, and enhances outer beauty. Water improves elimination, aids detoxification, and ends most cases of constipation (particularly when coupled with exercise). It aids the lymphatic system, adrenal glands and, of course, the kidneys. There's so much to love about water: It promotes excellent health and brings back the sparkle in your animal's eyes!

"But tap water, even most well water, is not the clean liquid your animal needs for good health....You have several choices to secure clean water. The best route is to invest in a home system that gives you a permanent source. Buying bottled water is an option, but it's unregulated, cumbersome, expensive and usually comes in plastic bottles. We have the most experience with distilled water . . . it works beautifully for all animals, regardless of health status or conditions . . . The beauty of distilled water at home is that it provides the *essence* of water—two parts hydrogen and one part oxygen, H_2O—and *that's all!* . . . We have a Pure Water brand [steam] distiller in our basement hooked directly to our plumbing (Call 800-875-5915 for a complete product and price list.) . . . The Doulton brand is [also] excellent . . . (Call 800-705-5559 for more information.)"

3. They strongly encourage owners to supplement their pets' diets with lecithin, biotin, vitamin E, and zinc. They give high marks to flaxseed oil, referring to it as "the Rolls Royce of oils" because it contains the greatest amount of essential fatty acids that contribute to "show-quality coats" every time.

The ABCs of Bathing

The Goldsteins believe that "hard-and-fast rules about bathing an animal are absurd!" The endless "debate over whether or not to bathe cats or a certain breed of dog is a [total] waste of time" since "a little soap or water never hurt any animal!"

Juliette de Baïracli Levy gave what I consider to be the "ultimate pet shampoo" for dogs and cats in her book *The Complete Herbal Book for the Dog* (see Appendix II). Here is the formula she used on her Afghan hounds with great success:

> First, bathe the pet with an oil-based (olive, flaxseed, vitamin E, Australian Tea Tree) soap. Then rinse away with rain water; if that isn't available then use distilled water. Now give the animal's coat *another* lathering. Only this time instead of using soap, use a homemade shampoo made by whipping up four farm-fresh eggs in a pint of warm water until the shampoo foams. Rinse this shampoo off the coat very well or it will adhere and spoil the fine shine that follows its proper use.
>
> For a final grooming shine, a "finish-off to grooming is friction and polishing" with a chamois cloth or old leather glove "dipped into cold common tea or a strong brew of rosemary herb. Or the bare hands can be dipped into the tea or herbal brew and used to polish the coat" that way.

You now have the information to turn an ordinary-looking cat or dog into a splendid and gorgeous creature that the world will admire and envy you for.

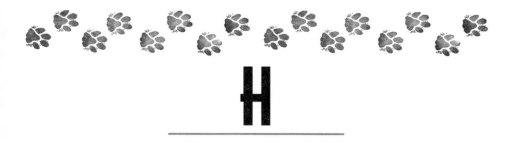

H

HAIR BALLS

A Frequent Problem in Cats

One problem commonly seen in longhair and medium-haired cats is the occurrence of hair or fur balls that result from frequent tongue grooming. Short-haired cats are also susceptible to it sometimes, but not as much as the other types are.

Normally, a cat should be able to cough up or discharge these frequent accumulations of hair without human intervention or assistance. I recall when my cat Jake resided in our former offices he would periodically bring up and leave hairballs deposited in different rooms of our Anthropological Research Center. At first I was puzzled by what they were, but I quickly learned of their origins when he spit one up one day while sitting in my lap, of all things.

The Cat Lady of Long Beach

I recently got a 7:30 A.M. Mountain Time wake-up call from Helen Steinmetz, aged 80, of Long Beach, California. She had a few questions relative to some things I mentioned in one of my books *(Heinerman's Encyclopedia of Nuts, Berries, and Seeds)*. After answering them to her satisfaction, I mentioned my then current writing project, namely this book.

This prompted her, in return, to relate some things she had been doing for her *many* cats. (She was always very coy and never disclosed the *actual* number she had.) "I give my cats liquid chlorophyll every day," she said. "I just pour some in their drinking water until it turns an emerald green and then let them have as much of it as they want to." But she did this only for those kept indoors. "For my outdoor cats, I just let them eat a little lawn grass or some sprouted wheat grass I clip and put out for them."

She claimed that since doing this, "None of them have ever had any problems with coughing up or discharging their hair balls." She said the veterinarians she had taken her pets to for this problem, "used things I didn't like to believe were natural." She made reference to Petromalt, Laxatone, and Laxaire, in particular, which come in paste form and are pushed down a cat's throat with a finger or tongue depressor.

Helen mentioned that the chlorophyll also kept her cats' bowels regular. "I feed them chicken and tuna once a day. I add a few drops of grapeseed and flaxseed oils to these canned-food mixes, which helps keep their coats shiny and sleek. I also give them enzymes by opening a capsule of Kyolic Formula 102 (see Product Appendix) and then adding this to the can of food. This is especially good for indoor cats."

She also believes in giving her cats a little liquid oxygen every day. "I add just two drops of DynamO$_2$ to their water. You have to be careful about how much is given at any one time, though," she cautioned. She spoke of how energetic these things made some of her older cats.

"Tony was my oldest cat. He passed on after 22 years of life. Even in his old age, he would continue moving about with the same grace and style that he did when he was only seven or eight." Other cats in her collection included Ginger ("a pretty little copper-red thing"), Rusty ("a very pretty red cat"), and Boy ("he's nearly twelve, I think, and has a gun-metal gray coat"). She takes in strays who are sick or injured and slowly nurses them back to health again. "I find it hard to turn one away when it comes to my door," she admitted. "I just have a 'soft spot' in my heart for cats," she openly confessed.

HEALTH CHECKUP

Becoming Your Vet's Assistant

Most medical doctors, hospital and life insurance groups, state and federal government agencies, and many companies in the business world routinely encourage or require their patients, members, or employees to submit to annual physical checkups. They do this in order to keep health costs down by detecting problems early on that can be treated less expensively.

In a similar fashion the same thing should be done with household pets. A pet owner becomes the eyes and ears of his or her veterinarian in between visits. The same care and attention given to preventive health in people should be routinely practiced with cats and dogs as well. By noticing something out of the ordinary, the pet owner can contact the vet and secure treatment before a serious problem develops.

Being aware of what is normal for a pet is the real key to noticing any unusual behavior or bodily changes. Thus, a monthly health check can assist the owner in focusing on a pet's good health rather than on a search for disease. Much of it is plain common sense, noted James Sokolowski, DVM, PhD, "but it can help an animal live a lot longer and certainly reduce veterinary bills."

He developed a five-point health check for household pets, although it can be applied to many other types of animals with some modifications. The procedure is simple. Dr. Sokolowski believes that a pet owner should handle his or her animal normally during the process, but give closer heed to it as he or she systematically checks it over from front to back and top to bottom. And what if the pet proves to be uncooperative? No problem, claims Dr. Sokolowski. Just employ some stealth and cunning and conduct the procedure without the pet ever suspecting what is going on. Be imaginative and try different things until you find out what is right and works for you, then do it.

5-POINT PET HEALTH CHECK

1. *Weight Check.* A pet needs to be weighed periodically just like its human master does. A cat should be weighed every four to six weeks at the same time and day of each month. One thing to bear in mind is that a major weight change doesn't need to occur in order to suggest there might be a problem. By standing above your pet and looking for a slight "waist" behind the animal's ribs, you will be able to detect any change in weight. Place both hands on the ani-

mal's ribs. You should be able to feel the ribs, but they shouldn't stick out, either. Also check for fat pouches in the groin area between the hind legs and beneath the stomach. Cats have a tendency to put on weight and become rather turnip-shaped.

2. *Coat and Skin Check.* Most pets have some kind of coat (except those genetically born without such). A cat's or dog's coat should feel uniformly smooth from head to tail when the hands are carefully run over or through it. Part the fur near the head and along the spine to check for flakes, scales, or cuts. Check for signs of fleas, including black flakes or specks, at the base of the tail and on the hindquarters and stomach.

3. *Eyes and Ears Check.* Gently pull down the lower eyelid to look for a pink color. The whites of the eyes should be glossy white with no redness. Look for normal pupil size and responsiveness of the pupil to light. Be on the lookout for a colored discharge, which could indicate possible infection. An animal's ears should appear clean, pink in color (not bright pink), and be free of debris and strong odors. Constant head shaking on an animal's part may suggest a buildup of dark wax or the presence of tiny ear mites.

4. *Teeth and Gums Check.* Lift your pet's lips away from its gums and press one finger gently but firmly over an upper tooth. When you remove your finger, the white color of the finger imprint on the gum should return to a natural, healthy pink color. Now open you pet's mouth to inspect all of its teeth. Beware of tartar buildup from commercial foods. This will be anywhere from yellow to dark brown in color.

5. *Spot Checks.* Scrutinize your animal carefully for unusual lumps or bumps by placing both hands on top of its head and moving down under the chin. Then move your hands behind the front legs, under the shoulders, down the back, over the hips, and down the legs. Inspect its claws and foot pads for cuts or cracks.

If you discover what may appear to be a potential problem or an out-of-the-ordinary change, be sure to contact your local vet to get a more accurate diagnosis. For instance, pets with dull or matted coats may not be getting the necessary nutrients they need. Poor diets may be at fault here, including consumption of commercial foods only. In that case, a pet's diet should be quickly adjusted to include more fresh foods (that is, *fresh* meat, *fresh* vegetables, and cooked *fresh* grains).

And make sure that your veterinarian has been apprised of any unusual lumps on the animal's body. Say, for instance, if you're running your hands over the pet's chest and abdominal area you discover an early mammary tumor that would otherwise be overlooked and go undetected until it was too late. Problems with a pet's eyes or ears also are important reasons to pay your vet a visit.

Just as it is with humans, "prevention is worth a pound of cure" when it comes to the health and well-being of your pet. Nothing compensates for detecting and preventing problems before they ever occur or get worse. Whatever time and effort you invest in your pet now, will be "money in the bank" and no anxiety in your mind later on.

(I am grateful to Susan Easterly for her ideas that contributed to this important section.)

HEART DISEASE

Canine Pacemakers

Pacemakers were first installed into human hearts in 1960. Some eight years later a few dogs started receiving their own versions. The first surgery happened at the University of Pennsylvania. Although this is an intricate operation, the implant procedure is surprisingly common. It has been estimated by one canine cardiologist that close to 300 pacemakers are put into dogs every year in America.

The pacemaker consists of a generator that is hermetically sealed inside a stainless-steel case. A plastic-covered wire lead comes out of the case and transfers an electrical impulse to a metal tip that touches the heart muscle, shocking it with each pulse.

The majority of canines receiving such instruments have shown signs of fainting due to slower-than-normal heartbeats. The two most common conditions are third-degree atrial-ventricular block and sick-sinus syndrome. Both result in a too-slow heart rate and periods where the heart might skip a beat for eight to ten seconds, which brings on a collapsing faint.

While the same generators are used in both humans and dogs, believe it or not the cost for the procedures differs drastically. The cost for humans is typically between $5,000 to $10,000 just for the device. My research-center staff administrator, Merrill Gee, had one of these inserted into his chest not long ago at a rather high price. Compare this to a mere $1,000 for a dog's *entire* procedure.

I watched one veterinarian insert such a device in the black Labrador of a friend of mine. The transvenous method was used, requiring just a tiny incision in the dog's neck. The surgeon placed the lead in the jugular vein, and using an X-ray machine that repeatedly took pictures of the lead's placement, advanced the lead all the way to the inside of the right ventricle. The generator was then placed beneath the skin, the lead was hooked to the generator, and the generator sent its electrical impulses to the dog's heart. This sure beats the old method of having to cut open the animal's chest and then actually screwing the tip of the lead directly into the heart before tunneling the lead to the outside.

I'm not one for surgery of any kind, mind you, but if an owner feels that his or her dog may need something like this, then it's nice to know what's affordable as a less invasive surgical alternative.

Herbs for the Heart

The three best herbs to give an animal for any type of heart disease are hawthorn berry, cayenne pepper, and garlic. They should be given in fluid extract or tincture form, as liquids are much easier to get down an animal than capsules or tablets are. This herbal trio should be used in succession and *always together* for maximum benefit. Mix in a small dish ten drops of hawthorn, four drops of capsicum, and six drops of liquid aged-garlic extract from Japan. Then fill an empty eyedropper with this mixture by holding the base to the liquid and then squeezing the rubber top part and letting it out again. Do this a couple of times until all of the liquid is inside the glass dropper. Then have someone else hold open the mouth of your dog or cat and squirt the fluids in toward the back of the throat. Do this every day.

Exercise Important

Animals, like people, need sufficient exercise in order to keep all their internal organs functioning properly. Dogs that have a nice big backyard can at least get some exercise every day to keep their weight down and stay in shape. For many other canines, though, this is a luxury that their apartment- or condominium-dwelling owners may not be able to afford. In such cases the owners are obligated to walk their dogs as often as they can—at least once a day for 30 to 45 minutes. In large cities such as New York there are professional dog walkers who are hired by pet owners to walk their dogs for an hour every day. When I've been to the Big Apple on media business related to the promotion of some of my new book titles, I've had several opportunities to see them in action. Usually there will be anywhere from 8 to 12 dogs *or more* all being walked at the same time. Once I even counted 18 dogs, but it was clear that the hapless walker was way in over his head and had more than he could handle. Still, it was amusing watching these different species of pooches making a complete fool out of him with their canine antics.

Healthful Heart Snacks

Both dogs and people love to snack on anything they rate high as edible munchies. The way to a dog's heart, both literally and figuratively, is to feed it homemade biscuits. I've collected several recipes that will be a treat for your pooch. Be careful, though, not to leave them in plain sight of your friends or relatives, who may mistake them for the real thing.

I'm indebted to Debbie Daniels-Zeller of Lynnwood, Washington, for creating these treats for her five healthy basset hounds. She writes: "You don't need Canine Biscuits 101 to make your own heavenly treats. You do need a basic plan to get the initial process down. Look at the ingredient options and how they work in recipes. First, your aim should be to mix up a consistent dough, though the taste and texture may vary. The dough should be easy to handle without being too sticky, yet not fall apart from too much flour. Once you've got them down, you can begin experimenting, doing variations and scanning your own favorite recipes for ideas.

"Biscuit recipes always include two essential parts: dry ingredients and wet ingredients, which are usually mixed separately, then combined. Following is a basic biscuit recipe, but the kind of flour, liquids and flavorings can always be changed to suit your dog's particular health needs or tastes. *Any* recipe can be altered once you understand what you're aiming to do."

ROSEMARY AND GARLIC BISCUITS

2½ cups whole wheat flour

½ cup ground sunflower seeds

1 teaspoon kelp

1 teaspoon rosemary

2 eggs, beaten

½ cup chicken stock

1 teaspoon liquid Japanese aged-garlic extract

or

2 cloves garlic, pressed

Combine all the dry ingredients, mixing well. Then combine the wet ingredients next until well-blended. Now mix both types of ingredients together, adding more liquid if necessary to form a stiff dough that can be formed into a ball by hand. (Debbie generally mixes the dough with her hands.) Set the dough aside for 30 minutes or cover and refrigerate a few hours or overnight if you wish.

Once the dough is chilled, preheat the oven to 350 degrees.

Roll the dough out to one-quarter-inch thick and cut it into shapes. The dough may be gathered up and rolled out again if necessary. You may crowd the biscuits onto the baking sheet if need be. Bake for 30 minutes. For a firmer biscuit, turn off the oven and let them sit until the oven is cool. You should get anywhere from four to eight dozen, depending on the size of biscuit cutter used.

Doggie Biscotti

3 eggs, well beaten
½ cup unsweetened applesauce
1 cup chicken stock
1 teaspoon liquid Japanese aged-garlic extract

or

2 cloves garlic, pressed
2 cups Arrowhead Mills kamut flour
1 cup millet flour
1 cup ground sunflower seeds
2 teaspoons aluminum-free baking powder
1 teaspoon kelp

(Note: See the Product Appendix under Wakunage for Japanese aged-garlic extract called for in both recipes.)

Mix the wet ingredients together. Then do the same with the dry ones, though separately. Spend a few minutes stirring everything so they get well blended. Next combine both wet and dry materials, adding flour or more liquid to make the dough stiff enough to handle, yet still slightly sticky.

Preheat the oven to 350 degrees.

Form the dough into three rolls, about 14 inches in length and lay them on one baking sheet. To keep the dough from sticking to your hands, slightly oil your hands with olive oil. Bake for close to 30 minutes. Take from the oven and let them cool for 15 minutes on a wire rack.

Now reduce the oven temperature to 325 degrees. Slice the biscotti on a slant, about one/half inch per cookie. Lay the biscotti flat on a cookie sheet and bake for another half hour or until dry. Turn off the oven and let the cookies cook in the oven for a harder biscotti. This makes more than 70 biscotti. Freeze to retain freshness.

Variations to this basic biscotti recipe can be made. Instead of the millet flour, you can use one-half cup each of wheat-grass and barley-grass powder. (See the Product Appendix under Pines.) It may take a little experimenting to get the dough just right, but the addition of both cereal grasses will give your dog more energy and help its heart and circulatory system a great deal.

The garlic, kelp, and rosemary in the first recipe are all antioxidants and excellent for preventing free-radical damage to the canine heart. You can work in a little powdered hawthorn berry, which is excellent for improving cardiac functions. All it takes is a little imagination, some patience, and a bit of experimentation to get things just right.

Calling All Hearts: Use Vitamin E Regularly

Over many years a significant amount of medical and veterinary research has demonstrated time and again that vitamin E is, without question, one of the best nutrients for preventing and treating existing heart disease in humans and animals alike. Because it is such a strong antioxidant, vitamin E can greatly reduce the amount of damage that delinquent molecules known as free radicals can do to heart-muscle tissues.

Various medical and veterinary journals have reported in times past that people and pets who consumed a minimum of 100 IU a day of vitamin E had an almost 50 percent lower risk of developing heart problems. Vitamin E enables animal and human hearts to beat more efficiently. It also prevents the "carmelization" of muscle tissue and body collagen, an intriguing aging process more properly known as glycation. Scientists working with animal and human models have discovered that two essential elements in these body tissues, protein and sugar, can also be harmful. They bind together under the body's own heat. The result is a kind of brown, molecular glue that attracts other proteins, gradually gumming up vital organs, including the eyes.

To better help the average reader understand what I mean by this, imagine yourself holding a metal measuring cup in which has been placed a mixture of egg yolks and milk (protein) and a little white sugar. Now hold it over a gas range and visualize in your mind what happens: The surface turns dark and stiff and sticky. Over time, that is exactly what happens to proteins in the animal or human body. Stuck together like this, they can cause harder arteries, stiffer joints, cataracts, and poor circulation.

One of the great contributing factors to this "carmelization" effect is the food we eat and that we feed to our pets. Much of this food is high in fat and sugar and has obviously been cooked. So we and our animal companions are ingesting stuff that has already been browned and carmelized without ever knowing it. In the process we are actually accelerating the aging syndrome in ourselves and our pets alike.

Vitamin E, of course, dramatically helps to reverse this trend. But drastic dietary changes are just as necessary. The inclusion of more fiber, the exclusion of fats and sugars, and the consumption of more *raw* or undercooked foods reduce any "carmelization" by 85 percent or better. The best vitamin E for accomplishing this won't be found in any health-food store or from any animal products company. But rather, it comes in a potent, totally unprocessed, animal-strength wheat-germ oil sold under the brand name of Rex. (See Product Appendix under Anthropological Research Center for more information.) Cats need around 200 IU daily, and dogs should be receiving 400 IU. My family and I have been taking a tablespoon of this liquid vitamin E for the last 30 years as well as giving it to our farm animals and past household pets with good results. We seem to be more limber and feel younger, as do our animals.

One Vet's Nutritional Plan for Cardiomyopathy

Dr. Bob Goldstein practices holistic veterinary medicine out of the Northern Skies Veterinary Center located in Westport, Connecticut. Bob was kind enough to let me include his nutritional plan for cardiomyopathy in this book. As he defined it in the September 1996 issue: "[This is] a disease of the muscular wall of the heart [and] can be caused by a poor diet. More cats suffer from [it] than dogs because of their bodies' high demand for amino acids.

"In my practice, I usually support animals with the L-carnitine and of course taurine (a deficiency in this amino acid has been linked to cardiomyopathy). I also recommend the supplements noted [following]. The co-enzyme Q10 supports energy production at the cellular level and is available in health-food stores. The Myocardial Drops help strengthen the heart muscle and Cardio Complex supports healing and blocks the body from causing further inflammatory degeneration. These supplements are available only through veterinarians from Professional Health Products (800-929-4133).

Nutrient Plan for Cardiomyopathy

This nutrient plan works in conjunction with conventional therapies. Show this nutritional plan to your conventional and holistic veterinarians and work [with them] to devise [something] that is suited to your cat's or dog's specific needs.

CATS AND SMALL DOGS (-12 LBS.)

L-carnitine—250 mg./daily
Co-enzyme Q10—10 mg./daily
Cardio Complex—½ tablet twice daily
Myocardian Drops—3 drops twice daily

MEDIUM DOGS (15-35 LBS.)

L-carnitine—500 mg./daily
Co-enzyme Q10—20 mg./daily
Cardio Complex—1 tablet twice daily
Myocardian Drops—5 drops twice daily

LARGE DOGS (50-85 LBS.)

L-carnitine—500 mg./daily
Co-enzyme Q10—40 mg./daily
Cardio Complex—1½ tablets twice daily
Myocardian Drops—7 drops twice daily

GIANT DOGS (85+ LBS.)

L-carnitine—750 mg./daily
Co-enzyme Q10—50 mg./daily
Cardio Complex—2 tablets twice daily
Myocardian Drops—10 drops twice daily

HEAT STROKE

Words of Advice from a Couple Who Care

Dr. Bob and Susan Goldstein have a deep and abiding love for animals. That is apparent to anyone who has been around them or taken the time to know them. He is a licensed vet and she is a trained animal nutritionist.

In the May 1996 issue of their newsletter, they carried a timely article on heat prostration from which confined animals may suffer. They strongly urge owners to *never* leave pets in closed vehicles, even if the window is down and they are parked in the shade. "A closed car on a warm day can reach 160° F. Dogs and cats do not have sweat glands to control overheating. They can cool down only by panting. Breathing hot air defeats the body's effort to cool down. Brain damage occurs when the body temperature reaches 106–107° F.

"Symptoms of heat prostration include: warm foot pads, glazed eyes, heavy panting, rapid pulse, deep red or purple tongue, high temperature, dizziness, vomiting, or diarrhea.

"Resist the temptation to leave your animal in the car. Our policy is never leave a dog, cat, or bird unattended in a car during the spring, summer or fall months.

Here are some worthwhile first-aid tips from them on how to treat heat stroke in confined animals:

1. Find people to help you. If it's a large- or medium-sized dog, enlist two volunteers. Have someone call the police and local veterinarian while you and the other volunteer move the animal to a shady area.

2. Move the dog to a cool shady spot. If needed, improvise a stretcher using a blanket or towel.

3. Splash cold water on the head, neck and extremities. If the water supply is limited, go to the head first and then the extremities. If ice is available, rub it on the gums or pack the paws in ice. Be careful around the mouth because an animal in distress may bite.

4. Administer a few drops of Rescue Remedy onto the tongue." [*Note:* Rescue Remedy is one of the most popular of the Bach-flower remedies, available in most health-food stores. For a full discussion of this item see the entry Trauma.]

Hip Dysplasia

A Common Skeletal Disease

In veterinary clinics the world over, one of the most frequently seen skeletal diseases in dogs is hip dysplasia. The problem appears to have a breed predilection—large-breed dogs, including Saint Bernards, German shepherds, Labrador retrievers, golden retrievers, and rottweilers. Smaller-breed dogs may be similarly affected, but are usually less likely to demonstrate clinical signs of it.

By clinical definition this disease is the malformation and degeneration of the coxofemoral joints. The systems most affected are the musculoskeletal. Considerable evidence points to its being a problem largely determined by an interaction of both genetic and environmental factors. Rapid weight gain, poor nutrition, and acquired pelvic muscle mass also influence the expression and progression of hip dysplasia.

The most common identifying markers are reduced activity, difficulty rising, reluctance to run or jump or climb stairs, intermittent or persistent hind limb lameness (often worse after exercise), "bunny hopping" or swaying gait, and narrow stance in the hind limbs. In more extreme situations, as I once saw in Dallas, Texas, in the early 1980s at a home of a friend, the afflicted animal (in this case a beautiful German shepherd) dragged his hind quarters around on the lawn and was unable to utilize his back legs at all.

Hip dysplasia begins in the immature dog. Clinical signs may become evident after only four months of age in some breeds of dogs. But other dogs may show the same clinical signs at an older age. Either way, the disorder can become very painful and distressing for the poor animal. Commercial dog food is suspected of inducing this in a number of instances.

A Beautiful Recovery

Cheryl Parker of Glendale Heights, Illinois, shared this particular story some 20 years ago. It offers hope for many others whose dogs are beginning to show clinical manifestations of the disease in its *earliest* stages.

"My five-year-old cocker spaniel had been suffering for over two months with a mysterious lameness. I took it to my vet who ran some tests but could find no reason for the problem.

"He was about to prescribe a potent muscle relaxant, but I stopped him from doing this. For it suddenly occurred to me that an article I had just read a few days before this mentioned the healing wonders of alfalfa. It was an article written by yourself [meaning me]. In it you explained how helpful it had proven to be in sports medicine in treating muscular aches and pains in humans.

"So I decided to give it a try on my pet. I fed my spaniel three alfalfa tablets daily. I crushed them into powder with a hammer and mixed them in with his regular food. I did this for a couple of weeks before his limping entirely disappeared. I relayed this to my veterinarian, who was astonished by the success I had had with it. Since then he as prescribed it to owners of countless other dogs suffering from hip dysplasia. But he has them add two emptied capsules of yucca powder with the alfalfa. Every *single* dog got well and walked again without further difficulties!"

A Dietary Approach

For many years most veterinarians never made a dietary connection to the problem of canine hip dysplasia. They usually informed pet owners that it was incurable and treated suffering animals with steroids, nonsteroid anti-inflammatory drugs (NSAIDS), and analgesics to reduce the severe pain and inflammation. For those who could afford it, hip-replacement surgery that cost several thousand dollars per hip was often recommended. Until only recently, hip dysplasia had pretty much been a death sentence for most canines.

Fortunately for pet owners, a new generation of veterinarians have begun taking a more holistic approach to the matter. They have placed nutrition first and focused on the dog's diet. They have counseled pet owners that feeding their canines processed commercial diets are placing such animals at high risk for this disease. Diets comprised largely of meat and poultry by-products with additional chemical preservatives, dyes, and fillers are especially notorious for inducing such a crippling animal disorder.

Instead, they have opted for more natural diets consisting of whole grains, meat, and vegetables (preferably raw, whole, and organically grown). Such holistic-minded vets have encouraged pet owners to give their canines antioxidants, vitamins B-complex, C, and D (if necessary), amino acids, and trace minerals. Dosages depend a lot on an individual dog's size, age, activity level, general health, and X-ray results, if these things are to be administered in supplement forms. (Consult the Product Appendix under Naturally Vitamins and Trace Minerals Research for reliable and trustworthy products that will be of assistance here.)

A friend of mine, Jerry Olarsch, a retired naturopathic physician in Florida, once told me how he restored the health and functioning of the dysplastic hips in his eight-year-old German shepherd. "I made sure she had fresh vegetables in her diet all the time. My wife and I would dice *raw* carrots or celery and include it with other things. I sprinkled some calcium-magnesium citrate powder into her food as well. Our dog was also given an electrolyte solution in her water to help assimilate the calcium better." The animal, which a conventional veterinarian had diagnosed as having severe dysplasia and for which he had recommended drug therapy, lived to the age of 16 without any further movement restrictions. In terms of doggie years and her previous condition, this was quite an incredible feat of achievement.

Every pet owner should take the time to study and prepare those types of foods, which can furnish their dogs with necessary nutrients that will either prevent or reverse hip dysplasia. By using some creative imagination, a number of delicious recipes can be created that dogs will enjoy chowing down and for which they'll be barking for for seconds. The following table shows which foods are highest in the necessary nutrients for this problem.

Antioxidants	Vitamins	Amino Acids	Trace Minerals
Broccoli	Beef liver	Beef (round steak)	Beans (black)
Carrots	Cottage cheese	Chicken	ConcenTrace*
Kale	Rice (brown)	Eggs	Fish (tuna in water)
	Yogurt (plain)	Fish	Lamb
		Oatmeal	Molasses
		Turkey	Potato
			Tofu
			Wheatgrass**

* Consult Product Appendix under Trace Minerals Research.

** Consult Product Appendix under Pines International.

Acupuncture Therapy

Acupuncture is an ancient therapy from China involving the judicious placement of needles at specific sites along nerves' pathways to evoke positive healing action and bring relief from distress and suffering. In modern times it has been medically validated and found to be extremely useful in very painful situations. Some holistic veterinarians have begun to incorporate modified versions of it into their own practices.

Such a person has been Allen M. Schoen, DVM, in Sherman, Connecticut. He uses it a lot to promote better circulation, reduce overall inflammation, and to provide local pain relief. Since acupuncture automatically promotes the release of endorphins into the animal's body, a canine previously in great pain and unable to rest can now relax and fall asleep thanks to these naturally generated body opiates.

Another practitioner using the same therapy to treat hip dysplasia and arthritis in animals is Terry Durkes, DVM of Marion, Indiana. Besides just using needles to stimulate various nerve points on the animal's body, he has developed a novel technique of permanently implanting tiny gold-plated beads beneath the skin so that the appropriate acupuncture points can be stimulated on a continuous basis. He prefers this treatment for young dogs with severe dysplasia that will need treatment their entire lives. Be advised, however, that this particular treatment is best suited for situations that produce a highly alkaline state in the body.

Massage and Manipulation

Still other holistic veterinarians approach the problem from different perspectives. One New England vet told me that he frequently massages canines to help reduce the pain and stiffness associated with hip dysplasia. "Ten minutes' worth of rubdown twice a day can break down fibrous tissue adhesions," he stated. "This expedites the removal of waste materials from the system and promotes more rapid healing." He usually has the owner standing beside the pet stroking face and head, while he concentrates on *lightly* massaging the bottom half of the animal. "A gentle touch is always needed here," he reminded me, due to the extreme pain felt by the canine.

Sue Ann Lesser, DVM, who practices her own version of veterinary chiropractic therapy on Long Island, New York, remarked that spinal manipulation gives dogs suffering from hip dysplasia more balance and physical comfort. She includes shark and bovine cartilage products and alfalfa meal in her treatment program, believing that these make the dog more responsive to spinal adjustments.

Herbs and Minerals

A growing number of holistic animal-care specialists are turning toward botanicals and ionic minerals to help relieve pain and joint stiffness in dysplastic and arthritic canines. These items often complement alternative therapies such as acupuncture, massage, and chiropractics. Especially helpful are anti-inflammatory plants such as alfalfa powder, flaxseed oil, liquid aged-garlic extract, marshmallow root, yucca, and licorice. (Consult the Product Appendix under Holistic Animal Care, Wakunaga of America, and Trace Minerals Research for additional information.)

A Case for The People's Court

Those who have watched some television in the last decade may recall the syndicated legal series, *The People's Court*. The idea originated in California some years ago with a simple premise: Take pending civil litigation, convince the litigants to waive their rights to a regular trial, persuade them to have their cases heard in a TV court forum, and be satisfied with whatever rulings were made by a retired judge. Just the notion of "*real* cases and *real* people" in an *actual* court of law, eventually garnered a wide audience, especially those who had grown tired of *Perry Mason* and other fictional television law programs.

Judge Joseph Wapner was the first TV judge and presided for many years, hearing numerous cases of every description. The producers eventually reformatted their program and took it to New York

City, where the retired mayor and former judge Edward J. Koch took over the bench and gavel pounding. The updated version includes audience participation from the Manhattan Mall (in which the show studio is located) and computer visitors to an interactive Web site. There are also three co-hosts, one of whom is a licensed and practicing attorney of many years. (In the original series there was only one host.)

One case that was televised recently on KSTU in Salt Lake City was appropriately entitled, "What will become of Rocky the Rottweiler?" The plaintiff, a traveling salesman by the name of Hakim, bought the dog from the defendant in March 1997. Finding that his dog walked with great effort, he consulted with two veterinarians who diagnosed the animal as having dysplasia in both hips. They told him it would cost $2,000 for a surgical correction to the problem or $195 to have the animal euthanized. He was suing to get back the $500 he had previously paid for the dog, plus other related expenses.

The defendant appeared along with the man who bred such dogs for a living. They maintained that the dog was okay at the time of sale and displayed no apparent walking disorders. They were upset with the prospect of the plaintiff selling Rocky to someone else in the condition he was in. They felt this was dishonest, given his present physical condition. They became further incensed in the courtroom upon learning from the plaintiff that he probably intended to have the rottweiler destroyed. The breeder agreed to take the animal back, get him prompt medical attention, and even pay for the operation out of his own pocket if necessary.

Judge Koch thought this was a very fair gesture. But then things took a sudden and unexpected turn: The plaintiff purposely hesitated to return the dog to the defendant and said he would have "to think it over" before making a decision. This further incensed the defendant and his friend. One of them shouted out, "You wouldn't want to be put to sleep if there was something physically wrong with you, would you?"

Judge Koch ruled in favor of the defendant, telling the plaintiff he had not made a strong enough case to show that the defendant was in the business of selling defective dogs. Nor had he proven with any evidence a case for fraud. "This was a private sale between two parties, and I have no choice but to rule in behalf of the defendant," the judge said. He then instructed Mr. Hakim, "You must decide whether to let the defendant's witness, the breeder, take the dog and find a good home for it and give it the proper medical attention it needs. Or to personally guarantee these gentlemen that you will have the operation performed on Rocky and not have him euthanized as you intimated doing earlier in this court."

Outside the courtroom stood one of the two male co-hosts with microphone in hand and cameras rolling, ready to interview the respective parties for brief summary comments as to how each one thought the trial proceedings went. But instead of civility, chaos and ugliness reigned. Bailiffs from the court had to rush out into the corridor and separate both parties before a nasty brawl started.

This authentic episode teaches two lessons. First, a viewer never knows what type of case will turn up on one of these TV court programs. And second, emotions run pretty high in people who truly love animals, and true resentment surfaces against their unnecessary destruction.

HOT SPOTS

One Pet Owner's Story

Hot spots are nothing more than a condition of wet eczema on the skins, ears, paws between the toes, and inside joints. It often is a sore eczema that has been infected. An itching rash and hot skin odor are fairly common. This is a condition common to vaginal and scrotal eczema.

The problem has been briefly dealt with in other sections of this book, most notably under Skin Problems. But one Illinois pet owner found a "sure-cure" treatment for her animal's hot spots. Here is her story.

Trudy Furstenberg has a two-year-old Lhasa apso, which developed a couple of hot spots on her hindquarters. She took her pet to a local animal clinic in the city of her residency, but left after discovering how much money they wanted to treat the condition. "The examination alone would have cost me $40," she exclaimed with some obvious irritation in her voice. "The full treatment would have been a lot more. I figured why pay them that kind of hard-earned money when I could probably do it myself."

She bought a few things from a pharmacy and health-food store before treating the dog herself. "First of all, I shaved away all of the hair around both areas, since that was contributing to the problem. Next, I sponged the bare skin with a small solution of distilled water and a little Palmolive dish detergent.

"Following this, I rinsed the areas clean with hydrogen peroxide," she continued. "I then sprayed the inflamed skin with a mixture of Inland Sea Water and fluid extract of goldenseal root. I mixed two tablespoons of the liquid herbal concentrate with one-half cup of the seawater and put it into a small spray bottle. The stuff worked really great. I applied it morning and night for ten straight days. After this, there was no more evidence of irritation. And just think, I probably saved myself a small fortune by doing so." (See Product Appendix under Trace Minerals for more information on Inland Sea Water.)

Holistic veterinarians frequently encourage their customers to put their pets on some kind of simple detoxification program to clear the problem up more quickly. They insist that, more often than not, a hot spot is only an external manifestation of an internal pollution situation. Putting the animal on a mild food or liquid fast (without meat) is one way. Also giving the afflicted pet daily doses of vitamin C (100 mg. for small sizes and double or triple that for larger sizes) helps as well. (For more ideas on detoxification see section under Cancer.)

"Russian Penicillin" Hits the Spot

The following true story from Lynn Allison came to me by way of Charlie Fox of Wakunaga in Mission Viejo, California.

"My beloved Lab, Jesse, came down with a nasty 'hot spot' on his back. I bathed the raw area, put triple antibiotic cream on the wound, and tried everything to help heal it. Unfortunately, Jesse managed to scratch it before a good solid scar could form and the 'hot spot' began to spread.

"I was researching the healing power of garlic during this time. I came across a testimonial from one pet owner who had applied liquid garlic from Japan topically to heal her pet's wound. And then I read about a Russian soldier who used garlic as a natural antibiotic to treat his gangrenous wounds with. I figured, 'What have I got to lose?' So, in desperation, I applied some of this 'Russian penicillin' from Japan on my dog's 'hot spot.' To my utter amazement the wound was nearly healed come the next morning! Jesse wasn't feeling itchy any more so he didn't have to scratch it open again. I was sold on this brand of garlic after that." (See Product Appendix under Wakunaga.)

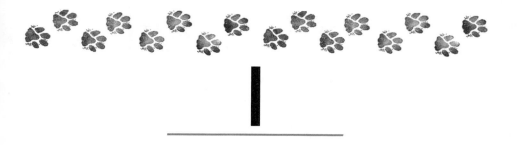

INFECTION

The Problem Defined

Over the years I've read a number of different books addressing the many health needs peculiar to humans and animals. While all of them referred to infection in general terms and some mentioned specific types, none actually defined the problem itself. I do so here because I feel it's important for the reader to understand the strange nature of infection in general.

Broadly speaking, an infection may be defined as an invasion and multiplication of microorganisms in the body tissues of man or beast. Such could be clinically inapparent or result in local cellular injury due to competitive metabolism, toxins, intracellular replication, or antigen-antibody response. The infection may remain localized, subclinical, and temporary if the human or animal body's defense mechanisms are effective. A local infection may persist and spread by extension to become an acute, subacute, or chronic clinical infection or disease state. A local infection could also become systemic when the microorganisms gain access to the lymphatic or vascular system.

The only exception to the foregoing definition would be the usual multiplication of "normal" bacterial flora of the intestinal tract. Such isn't viewed as an infection, but as an essential part of nature for promoting healthy bowel ecology. Only when such bacteria somehow manage to enter the bloodstream periodically do severe pathological consequences result.

As a rule, bacteria cause infection. They are unicellular prokaryotic microorganisms that generally multiply by cell division. They have cell walls that provide constancy of form. They may be oxygen-dependent (aerobic) or can live and grow in the absence of molecular oxygen (anaerobic). Bacteria may also have spontaneous movement (motile) or else be without it (nonmotile). Furthermore, they can be free-living, saprophytic (thriving on decayed organic matter), parasitic (growing in or on a living host), or pathogenic (disease-inducing).

Undiscerning and Apparent Manifestations

Invading bacteria produce toxins that damage host tissues and interfere with normal metabolism. Some of these toxins are actually enzymes that, by breaking down host tissues, prevent the localization of infections, thereby causing them to spread elsewhere in the biological system. Other bacterial substances destroy the host's immune-system scavenger cells (phagocytes) that are capable of ingesting bacteria, foreign particles, and other cells, if necessary.

Viruses are parasitic on host cells, induce cellular degeneration (as in rabies or AIDS), or cellular proliferation (as in warts or cold sores). Substances produced by many invading organisms cause allergic sensitivity in the host. The immune response to viral infection has been implicated in some diseases.

The body of a human being or animal has numerous mechanisms for protecting itself from bacteria or viruses. Intact epithelia act as a physical barrier, but once it has been penetrated, protective responses are activated in the underlying connective tissue proper. These are the inflammatory and immune responses. Inflammation is a nonspecific, local response that develops quickly and limits the damage to the injury site. The immune response, on the other hand, takes longer to develop and is highly specific. It destroys particular infectious microorganisms and foreign molecules at the site of infection and throughout the human or animal body.

Just about any infection will lead to an inflammatory response. As short-term or acute inflammation develops in connective tissue, it produces four symptoms: heat, redness, swelling, and pain.

The body of an infected person or pet wages an elaborate warfare against harmful bacteria and viruses. Every component conceivable within the immune arsenal is brought forth to bear against such microorganisms. The actual processes involved are lengthy and complicated and need not be detailed here. Suffice it to say, glandular enlargement, tissue swelling, pus accumulation, foul odor, and allergic reactions are typical manifestations of the immune response.

This, then, is essentially the anatomy of an infection in man or beast.

The Benefits of Natural Procedures

With the advent of World War II, the giant pharmaceutical industry found it necessary to invent and manufacture many different types of synthetic drugs to replace those natural substances formerly used. There were several incentives for doing so. First, they could be mass produced and, second, done so quite economically. They also were more specific and potent in their actions and worked more quickly than natural things did.

For a number of decades these chemical replacements efficiently served the health needs of men, women, and children as well as the animals they bred and raised for monetary purposes and pleasure. But then some odd things began happening along the way. The bacteria and viruses such drugs were intended to combat started getting smarter. As newer generations evolved, they developed increasing resistance to these medications, rendering them fairly ineffective in many instances.

As body systems became overwhelmed with such a vast array of synthetic pharmaceuticals, they soon rebelled in the form of toxic reactions. Such untoward side effects created special problems of their own above and beyond the infectious diseases themselves. In time many within the general population became highly suspicious and distrusting of most chemical drugs. They opted for natural approaches and went in search of the same for themselves and the animals they loved.

This brings us to the current state of affairs that much of our society is now in. Knowledgeable and thoughtful people everywhere have switched to alternative medicines in droves and pretty much abandoned the old ways and measures. Fortunately for themselves and their pets, it is no longer business as usual. What the orthodox medical doctor or veterinarian may continue to prescribe is being taken with many grains of salt these days. Disillusioned patrons have cast their attention in other directions in search of practitioners who use other methods and modalities that are considered safer and more natural.

For our purposes, the discussion on suitable remedies for managing infections will be confined to botanicals and nutrients. Their benefits are several and should be mentioned in passing. Probably the most significant feature to start with is that they can tackle even the most aggressive and stubborn drug-resistant bacteria and viruses, which even regular pharmaceutical agents can no longer adequately touch. Another thing is these natural substances are *living* materials and impart *life* to the human or animal body. Synthetic drugs are artificial and inert, having no real life in them. And they are usually quite safe and do virtually no harm to a biological system except to restore it to health.

The standard medications that have been used extensively by medical doctors and veterinarians for so long are at best good for combat and nothing else. Until only recently they still managed to do a fair job of containing enemy microorganisms. But they are like their counterparts of the Second World War, the Sherman tanks that battled Rommel's Nazi forces in North Africa or the B-17 Liberators and B-29 Fortresses that dropped bombs over Germany and Japan, that have long since been retired and replaced with more efficient fighting equipment.

So, too, must the old drugs be phased out and herbs and nutrients substituted for them. Natural agents not only stop the nefarious activities of harmful bacteria and viruses, but they also promote healing. That is to say, they *assist* the human or animal body to effectively *rebuild* itself. In this they go far beyond what the pharmaceuticals were capable of doing. And since they are life-giving to begin with, they can do this nicely, whereas the inert drugs can't do that.

Coping with Infection the Natural Way

In attempting to find natural solutions to complex problems that periodically change, it is important to rely on "broad-spectrum treatment" instead of a single therapy approach. This was reiterated several times by Steven W. Dow, DVM, of Fort Collins, Colorado, in his short treatise "Anaerobic Infections in Dogs and Cats," which appeared in *Current Veterinary Therapy: Small Animal Practice* (10th Ed.) (Philadelphia: W. B. Saunders Co., 1989; pp. 1082–85), edited by Robert W. Kirk, DVM. The chief reason for doing this, according to Dr. Dow, is that current strains of bacteria are usually highly resistant to first- and second-, sometimes even third-generation antibiotics. By using a mixture of several instead of just one, it keeps the bacteria from adapting so quickly to the drugs intended to kill them.

This matter of "mixing up" applies with equal force when utilizing natural antibiotic substances, such as garlic, goldenseal root, and Echinacea. Go back and read the first several pages of this entry regarding the unique behavioral characteristics of bacteria and viruses. These three herbs, better than anything else, are capable of fighting the worst kinds of anaerobic and viral infections that commonly beset dogs and cats. Each of these particular herbs contain different chemical constituents that disarm bacteria and viruses before they can cause further damage in the system of a pet. They are better as a team than when used independently.

In his own approach to the problem, Dr. Dow refers to a number of standard antimicrobials currently used in veterinary practice. Undoubtedly, he wasn't acquainted with alternative replacements from the botanical kingdom. But at least his tiered concept of drug administration makes a lot of sense, whether a veterinarian is staying with traditional medications or having the courage and vision to opt for safer and more natural remedies. By layering several botanicals into the system at once or within a 12-hour period every day, a sort of "biochemical chaos" is created amoung the harmful bacteria or viruses. Their progress is checked, they are denied the means to cause further havoc, and infection soon ceases.

One Dog Owner's Story

A female dermatologist from the East Coast was attending a conference on anti-aging at the Lexus Park Hotel in Las Vegas, Nevada, in December 1997. I happened to be there doing a book signing at the Calorad Team 21 Support Group exhibit when this woman happened to stroll by. She registered for a copy of my *Encyclopedia of Anti-Aging* (Englewood Cliffs, NJ: Prentice Hall, 1996), which was then being distributed free of charge.

She waited patiently in line until the chair beside the table I sat at became vacant. We shook hands, and I then thanked her for waiting so long. We laughed together when I mused aloud, "It's probably good for doctors like yourself to stand in line for a while, so they know how their patients feel when they keep them waiting for a long time." After several minutes of professional chit-chat on human health matters, the conversation turned to pets after I told her about this book I was then finishing for my publisher.

Being alternative-minded when it came to matters such as this, she told me a wonderful story of her own healing experience with garlic, goldenseal, and Echinacea. I believe it is worth repeating here, though she asked that neither her name nor the city of her residency and practice be used.

"About a month ago, I noticed that my French poodle, Fifi, was hobbling around on only three legs. I looked at her paw and discovered that one toe was seriously inflamed and quite tender to touch. I took her to an upscale veterinary clinic, and one of the best doctors there examined her more carefully. He gave her an injection and said she would be fine. But three days later that one toe had nearly swollen to about the size of her entire foot. Returning to the same clinic, the doctor in charge made a small incision to investigate the problem further. He discovered a small, pea-size lump, which he matter-of-factly declared had nothing to do with her suffering. Other than that he could find no other cause for the problem.

"He heavily medicated her paw and wrapped it up. I was given some medication—cefoxitin, I think it was—and requested to bring my dog back in a couple of days. Fifi continued to move only as necessary. I kept the next appointment and watched as the bandage was removed. The incision was open wide, exposing infected tissue, and the swelling had not decreased at all. The same veterinarian scratched his head in wonderment, almost as if to suggest that this was something they hadn't taught him in veterinary school.

"As a last resort, though, he wanted to surgically remove her whole toe, which was 'standard operating procedure for most dogs,' I was informed. Following the toe cutting, I was to put a clean sock over the foot to prevent her from licking the incision, continue with the antibiotic, and keep him informed of Fifi's progress. Right then and there, I decided enough was enough! I picked up my poodle without having the incision closed and marched right out of there with an angry and defiant attitude.

"I took my dog home and then went to a health-food store that carried an extensive line of liquid botanicals. I purchased the liquid form of Kyolic aged garlic and fluid extracts of goldenseal root and Echinacea. I thoroughly saturated a cotton ball with a mixture (15 drops) of all three solutions. I placed it over the incision for several minutes. I also dribbled some in the wound itself. Then I placed a clean sock over her foot. I also gave her some of the liquid combination mixed in with some beef broth to lap up." (*Note:* For cats, use some canned tuna fish or salmon oil or water when adding 15 drops of this herbal mixture). "I also gave my dog some vitamin C capsules (600 mg.).

"By the end of the third day the swelling showed evidence of subsiding. The incision was also starting to close up. By the fourth day, the incision was totally closed and the toe was almost its normal size. I took my dog back to the vet clinic on the sixth day and the head doctor was dumbfounded at the condition of the toe. After getting over the initial shock of surprise, he confessed with some trepidation that he probably didn't know everything there was to know about puzzling infections like this. He felt even more ashamed to know that a lady dermatologist had come up with a better solution than he had. But he did express pleasure in knowing that my remedies had worked.

"Strange to say, though, now that I think about it," my informant thoughtfully concluded, "he never did ask me for any further information about what I had done, beyond the fact that I had told him I had just used three herbs to make her well again. I guess this just goes to show that you can lead a horse to water, but not get him to drink."

Some Other Supplement Choices

Giving an infected pet daily doses of vitamin A (fish oil, 5,000 IU) and vitamin E (one teaspoon Rex's Wheat Germ Oil), as well as powdered or liquid vitamin C (about 500 mg.), enables a weakened immune system to fight infection more aggressively.

There are also two liquid herb preparations that are an immune stimulant and viral detoxicant. These should be used in conjunction with an ionic mineral concentration from the Great Salt Lake (ten drops of each mixed together). (Consult the Product Appendix for further information. For vitamins, look under Naturally Vitamins. For the wheat-germ oil, look under Anthropological Research Center. For the herbal-fluid extracts, look under Holistic Animal Care. And for the mineral ConcenTrace, look under Trace Minerals Research.)

Thinking Green for Rapid Recovery

A section of this size on infection wouldn't be complete without mentioning one other natural substance. In fact, I would almost be persuaded to say that if nothing else were used but plant chlorophyll in an infected dog or cat, that animal would recover of its own accord in sufficient time. I've worked with chlorophyll for many years in thousands of healing situations that involved both humans and animals. In *every single case* where chlorophyll was applied, either by itself or with other things, *total* healing and *complete* recovery ensued.

There are a number of different chlorophyll sources to draw from. Some of the best are celery, parsley, and endive. They make a terrific solution to bathe an infected wound with as well as for internal use. But getting it down is the tricky part. Flavoring some of this chlorophyll juice with a little beef or fish broth should satisfy the most timid dog or fussiest cat. (Use a Vita-Mix 5000 to obtain the necessary chlorophyll juice from the aforementioned leafy greens.)

Another wonderful source are certain cereal grasses that grow in the organic soil and cold winter climate of Lawrence, Kansas. A product called Mighty Greens is in my estimation *the* strongest source of mixed chlorophylls (grain, vegetable, and seaweed) that I've ever become acquainted with. Mixing one teaspoon of the powder in four ounces of spring water and six ounces of beef broth (dogs) or fish broth (cats) will definitely clear up the worst infection imaginable, even if nothing else is used. (Consult the Product Appendix under Vita-Mix Corp. and Pines International for more information on the items cited here.) (Also see Influenza.)

INFLUENZA

Give Your Animal "Nature's Flu Shot" During the Winter Months

Dr. Bob Goldstein and his wife are the editors and authors of the monthly newsletter *Love of Animals* (see Appendix II for subscription information). They gave their permission for the following data that was borrowed from their December 1996 issue to be reproduced here for a much larger and wider reading audience. "We do this for you, John," Bob said in a recent phone conversation from his home in Westport, Connecticut, "in the belief that it will do many others a lot of good."

"This recipe was passed on to us by a healer who wanted to keep this American Indian remedy alive. Even we didn't realize the power of this remedy until we began sharing it." The Goldsteins describe it as their version of "nature's flu shot." It is virtually impossible, they declare, for infectious viruses and bacteria to take hold and reside in an animal's system when this pure, mineral-rich drink is lapped up by household pets. "This broth gives you a healthier choice than automatically turning to antibiotics for respiratory infections.

They suggest making a batch of their broth ahead of when it's needed and then freezing small portions. "When you sense there's something brewing or you hear that first sneeze, pull it out and warm it on the stove. (Please avoid reheating the broth in a microwave because it changes the molecular structure of the minerals, making them less potent.)

"For an active infection, serve the broth alone as part of a 24 hour fast. Add the broth to cooked brown rice for another two or four meals. This will fill the body with healing minerals and pure water. Then return to regular feeding. You can use the same plan to soothe an arthritic flare-up.

"You can make this broth with just the potato skins and water for a potassium-rich drink." [*Note:* This would also be ideal for pet owners suffering from hypertension and renal problems.] To bring in other healing ingredients, try this deluxe version. We prefer organic ingredients whenever possible but you can use conventionally grown vegetables. [*Note:* I added just one ingredient to their recipe list, believing that it will greatly enhance the mineral content even more. Consult the Product Appendix under Trace Minerals for more information.]

POTATO PEELING BROTH

2 quarts filtered water
12–15 drops liquid ConcenTrace
8–10 medium potatoes, peel skin one-quarter-inch thick (discard core)
6 carrots, cut into 1 inch pieces (finely chop carrot tops if available)
6 celery stalks, cut into 1-inch pieces
3–4 cloves garlic, cut in half
1 tablespoon ginger root, rough slices
4 sprigs parsley

Peel the potatoes with heavy strokes, approximately one-quarter-inch thick. Put the peelings in a three-quart pot and cover with the filtered water. (Use distilled water for arthritic inflammation.) Add carrots, celery, garlic, ginger root, and parsley. Bring to a boil and simmer for one hour, covered. You may strain out the vegetables or feed with vegetables for a heartier soup. This recipe makes approximately a three-day supply for a medium-sized dog.

Strain out vegetables if freezing in small portions. Defrost one or two hours before serving or reheat to lukewarm over stove top.

DOSAGE PER MEAL

Cats and small dogs (1–12 lbs.)—½ cup
Medium dogs (15–35 lbs.)—1 cup
Large dogs (50–85 lbs.)—2 cups
Giant dogs (85+ lbs.)—3 cups

Vitamin C Is Health Insurance for Your Pet

The Goldsteins believe in the power of vitamin C to ward off colds and flu in humans as well as in the animals they adore. "It may not be flashy, but vitamin C can be a powerful health aid for you [in the winter].

"One drawback of this vitamin is that it can be tough on the digestive system. Boosting an animal's intake of vitamin C sometimes produces flatulence and loose stool. Those problems are solved by using a form of this vitamin called Ester C." They say they've "rarely heard complaints about it causing an animal discomfort" in all the years they've both been working with it. "Ester C is gentle because it is pH neutral.

"Introduce Ester C slowly. Start with one-quarter the recommended dose and double the amount every four days until the desired daily amount is reached. For small animals, do your best to eyeball the dosages. You do not have to be exact.

"The daily dosages [we] recommend for general good health are [follow]. Give once a day with food. If your animal is sick or has a chronic condition, double these amounts simply by giving with the A.M. and P.M. meals."

ESTER C FOR COLD AND FLU PREVENTION

Weight	Capsules or Tablets	Powder (4,600 mg/teaspoon)
Cats and small dogs (1–12 lbs.)	250 mg	1/16 teaspoon
Medium dogs (15–35 lbs.)	750 mg	1/8 teaspoon
Large dogs (50–85 lbs.)	1,500 mg	1/4 teaspoon
Giant dogs (85+ lbs.)	2,000 mg	1/2 teaspoon

(Also see Infection.)

ITCHING

Initial Signs

The act of scratching, licking, biting, or chewing are the most common signs of pruritus in cats and dogs. But in some animals one may have to look for evidence of self-inflicted trauma and skin inflammation in order to make a complete diagnosis.

Cat owners, in particular, should be made aware of something else. Their pets are notorious for being secret lickers. Hair loss without accompanying skin inflammation may be the only external manifestation of itching.

Different Factors Involved

Itching may be induced by a wide variety of things. The most common, of course, would be parasitic in origin. Into this group would fall fleas, scabies, lice, and so forth.

Allergies are probably the second biggest cause for itching. The pet could have a particular allergy to a specific parasite. Or it could suffer from an undisclosed food or drug allergy. The animal might also be experiencing a "bacterial hypersensitivity" that would require the services of a veterinarian to confirm with certainty.

Other miscellaneous factors include primary and secondary skin scaling, a phosphorus deficiency, skin cancer, immune-related disorders, and endocrine-gland dysfunctions. Their involvement with the itching varies considerably and may not always be discernible at first glance. A more thorough and professional diagnosis for them may be necessary.

The Psychological Aspect

For years most veterinarians treated animals without much regard to how they felt or what they thought. But we know from biblical literature (Revelation 4 and 5) as well as modern science (animal-behavior studies) that animals are endowed with wonderful reasoning capabilities that permit them emotions and ideas. Granted that their feelings and thoughts may not be on par with those experienced by human beings, but they are, nevertheless, genuine for their own species and should be accepted as valid.

Cats and dogs are especially highly sociable creatures. Helen Steinmetz (mentioned elsewhere in this book) of Long Beach, California, told me in a recent telephone conversation: "Cats [and dogs, for that matter, too] just love to be talked to. And hugged and petted and given attention just like anyone else would. They are really no different than us in that respect. My cats [she had a lot of them] won't even begin to eat until I've chatted with them a little and stroked them. They like this and respond very well to displays of affection."

A few psychologists who specialize exclusively in animal behavior have declared that animals can get just as bored, obsessed, upset, or depressed as any humans can. When this happens they may resort to excessive grooming, nervous behavior (manifested in spinning, tail chasing, imaginary air-fly biting, pacing, staring, self-directed vocalization, fabric sucking and chewing, and some aggressions), and inconsistent eating and sleeping patterns.

These things are believed to be responsible for what is known as psychogenic alopecia, when other factors have been ruled out. Hence, the psychological dimension needs to be given serious consideration when attempting to deal with a condition as general in scope as itching.

Herbal Therapy

Herbs work quite well in treating small-animal pruritus. But the choice of botanicals depends in large part upon what the cause of the problem is. For example, if fleas or lice (see individual sections) are discovered to be the culprits, then fluid extracts such as garlic, goldenseal, and wormwood (10-15 drops orally or in water) would be efficacious. The application of different oils such as eucalyptus, melaleuca, and tea tree oil definitely help, too.

If an allergic reaction to food or medicine is suspected, then a careful review of what is given the pet seems to be in order. The overfeeding of commercial canned or packaged foods and the overuse of some drugs are the cause of better than 85 percent of most animal itching. The administration of vitamin C (1,000 mg.), B-complex (high potency), and brewer's yeast in the food supply have proven to be extremely useful in controlling allergies.

A few mineral deficiencies should be ruled out as another likely cause for animal pruritus. I've discovered that adding ten drops of liquid ionic mineral concentrate from the Great Salt Lake to an animal's water each day will help to stop any itching that may be due to a lack of specific minerals. (See the Product Appendix under Nature's Answer, Naturally Vitamins, and Trace Minerals Research for information on how to obtain the items mentioned here.)

Witch-hazel tincture, which can be purchased at any supermarket or drugstore, is a good across-the-board remedy for relieving itching in general. And so is peppermint tea. Either one can be put into a spray bottle and squirted directly on the animal's skin for quick relief. They are safe and effective to use.

Have You Hugged Your Pet Lately?

Last but not least, it should be remembered that animals are divine creations possessed with spirits or souls just as we are, but obviously on a different level of reasoning and feeling capabilities. They get lonely, frightened, angry, and lose interest just as we do.

They are no different from us in the need for attention. Frequent hand pats to the head or face, back and side stroking, hugging, arm cradling, and carrying on one-sided conversations are all excellent therapies toward greatly motivating distraught pets. When enough of this is done, the animals' psychogenic itching should disappear pretty quickly.

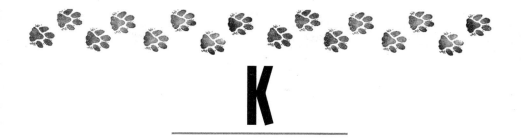

K

KIDNEY FAILURE

Natural Treatment that Works from a Holistic Veterinarian

Dr. Robert S. Goldstein has a treatment program from renal disease that is unique to his holistic expertise. He granted permission for the following data to be copied for use in this text for the benefit of my readers. I'm grateful, as always, to him and Susan for this. This piece appeared in the January 1997 issue of *Love of Animals.*

"Kidney failure is the second leading cause of death among cats. An estimated 25 percent of dogs have some form of the disease. The tough part about kidney disease is that animals may not show signs for months, even years. The damage is usually advanced by the time symptoms surface—excessive thirst, weight loss, poor appetite, vomiting, the smell of urine on the skin and in the mouth.

"(I urge you to uncover health problems such as kidney disease early by taking your dog or cat in for an annual physical examination.)

"Conventional medical therapy generally consists of fluids intravenously or subcutaneously to flush the body. Antibiotics and cortisone address secondary symptoms such as nausea, vomiting and loss of appetite. In contrast, the holistic approach asks, 'Why have the kidneys stopped working?' Therapy then focuses on relieving inflammation in the kidneys and strengthening them and the other internal organs.

"The combination of approaches—the medical to stabilize the acute internal poisoning and the holistic to strengthen the internal organs—usually improves the animal's quality of life and, in many

191

cases, extends their life. Years ago, I was shocked to learn on a routine blood test that my own Doberman, Christy, had developed acute renal failure.

"In a standard blood test, the Blood Urea Nitrogen, or BUN, measures how well the kidneys are filtering the waste created from the breakdown of proteins. An elevated BUN level is an indication that the kidneys are not operating up to par. Normal BUN levels range from 8 to 25 for dogs and 10 to 35 for cats. At a BUN level of over 200, Christy had weeks to live, according to my conventional training.

"Along with my brother Marty, who also is a holistic veterinarian, I first stabilized the blood poisoning with intravenous fluids, a standard conventional approach. (I did enhance the intravenous fluids with vitamins, which I wish other veterinarians would do.) After she was stable (BUN in the 50 to 60 range), we began an oral program of nutritional glandular and homeopathic remedies. This therapy is what most animals do not receive from a conventional veterinarian, but it held her blood level in a reasonable range. Christy lived for another 13 months and for 12 of those months, she was a happy, care-free dog. The only differences in her life were many supportive remedies and a diet lighter in protein.

"In my practice, I treat more cats with kidney disease than I do cats with cancer. With dogs, my patients are about 3-to-1 cancer to kidney disease."

His nutritional program, though not given in detail, includes a glandular (bovine liver) supplement and vitamin-B complex (either as brewer's yeast or in a formula mixture). His Alternative Kidney Diet supplies other needful nutrients in food forms. "Missing from most diets is consideration of the quality of the protein," he continued. "If you're interested in cooking once in a while for your pet, a healthy recipe such as the one [following] nourishes the system, without taxing the kidneys.

"My kidney diet may be served solo as an alternative to pet food or may be mixed with any natural, low protein food of your choice. If you like, you may vary the grains by feeding oatmeal or barley. Parsley and asparagus work as gentle diuretics helping the kidney flush wastes and impurities. Also, for dogs you may occasionally substitute tofu for the chicken."

Dr. Bob's "Kidney" Mix

1 cup brown rice or millet
3 cups filtered water
2 raw egg yolks (organic)
½ cup cubed, deboned chicken meat (hormone and antibiotic free)
2 tablespoons chopped parsley
2 tablespoons grated asparagus
1 tablespoon sesame oil (unrefined)

Cook rice (or millet) well with two-and-a-half cups water, approximately 45 minutes. In remaining one-half cup of water, cook cubes of chicken (about five minutes). Mix chicken and grain with chopped raw vegetables and oil. When cooled, add egg yolks, multivitamin, and other supplements to mixture. If your animal's appetite is poor, flavor the stew with plain, organic nonfat yogurt (2 teaspoons for cats and one-and-a-half tablespoons for dogs).

As Meal:

Small dogs (1–12 lbs.)—¼–½ cup
Medium dogs (15–35 lbs.)—1 cup
Large dogs (50–85 lbs.)—2 cups
Giant dogs (85+ lbs.)—2–3½ cups

Nutritional and Herbal Assistance for Cats

In the preparation of this book, I had frequent occasions to interview holistic and some nonholistic veterinarians around the country whose knowledge and expertise I respected. I discovered that there were just as many varied opinions and methods of treatment as there usually are in regular medical care for people. Doctors in both systems of medicine, while trained pretty much the same in the basic stuff, each develop their own way of approaching specific problems. Thus, no two veterinarians will treat renal disease exactly alike in a sick cat. Granted that there may be overlapping similarities, but generally speaking there will also be quite noticeable differences.

In gathering together an assortment of nutritional and botanical modalities, I picked out those deemed to be the most sensible, discarded what I didn't care for (such as homeopathic preparations), and added a few things of my own that I knew work well in such situations. I am grateful to Dr. Shannon Hines of the Orchard Animal Clinic in Bountiful, Utah, for valuable input. She graduated from the Oregon State Veterinary Medical College in Corvallis and has been in regular practice for almost eight years (with about two-and-a-half years of that in holistic therapy alone).

Dr. Hines said it is easier to dispense liquid preparations into felines than giving them either capsules or tablets. "You take the cat by the scruff of its neck and hold the head back," she advised. "The mouth automatically opens (in most instances) and you can squeeze the liquid in that way" without getting scratched or bitten. If the mouth doesn't open all the way, there will be enough of a space at the corners into which a dropper can be put and the fluids squirted out.

FELINE FORMULA FOR KIDNEY FAILURE

THE TEA PORTION

1 pint of spring, purified, or distilled water
¼ teaspoon stinging nettles
¼ teaspoon alfalfa
¼ teaspoon red raspberry
¼ teaspoon dandelion root/leaves
¼ teaspoon cornsilk
¼ teaspoon cleavers
8 drops liquid ConcenTrace (see Product Appendix under Trace Minerals)

Add the ConcenTrace drops to the water before boiling it. Then the dandelion root and leaves. Cover with a lid, reduce heat, and simmer 4 minutes. Set aside, remove lid, and add rest of ingredients. Cover and steep 30 minutes. *Note:* It is better to use the crude, coarsely cut, and dried herbs to make this tea than their powdered equivalents. Strain and set tea aside.

(continued)

The Nutritional Mix Part

⅛ teaspoon bee pollen
⅛ teaspoon powdered kelp
¼ teaspoon wheat grass
¼ teaspoon barley grass
¼ teaspoon cod-liver oil
¼ teaspoon Rex Wheat Germ Oil
¼ teaspoon liquid lecithin

In a blender combine the strained tea liquid and the other ingredients in their given order. Run the machine for two minutes with the lid securely locked in place. Stop the unit and check the material; it should be rather runny. If not, add a little more pure water until it becomes sufficiently liquefied.

Strain through a fine wire-mesh strainer or double-layered cheesecloth. Store in a dark amber bottle in the refrigerator. *Shake well* before using each time as contents are apt to separate or settle. Pour into a clean cup only that amount to be used for the day and return the rest to the refrigerator. Allow the liquid to set at room temperature for a while until it becomes lukewarm.

Using a syringe or turkey baster, fill with a little of the liquid (no more than ¾ teaspoon at a time) and insert into the cat's mouth. Repeat twice daily, morning and evening.

Taurine and potassium are also critical nutrients for felines with kidney problems. Fish protein is high in this sulfur-bearing amino acid (sardines and mackerel are good sources). Banana is high in potassium: Liquefy ¼ peeled banana with ⅔ tablespoons of mineral water in a blender and give to cat same way as you would my other formula.

Kidney Stones

A Painful Affliction

The proper medical term for this disorder is renal (kidney) calculi (from the Latin term for "pebble"). These are abnormal concentrations occurring within animal or human bodies that are generally composed of mineral salts. They can be extremely painful to pets and their masters alike.

Veterinary medicine has its own special designations for this problem. Kidney stones in cats are known as struvite uroliths. They occur in both the upper and lower urinary tracts.

The same name applies for kidney stones in dogs. These are usually brought on by excessive consumption of dietary protein and only moderate intakes of water. Genetics plays a bigger role in their formation in some breeds of dogs than it does in cats. Miniature schnauzers and English cocker spaniels are particularly susceptible to sterile struvite uroliths. And, as in cats, both the upper as well as the lower portions of the urinary tract are adversely affected.

Kidney stones in small animals cannot be dissolved. *But* they can be passed out of the system through natural means. More often than not, owners elect for surgery, which can be traumatic to any animal.

British Herbs to the Rescue

Some years ago when I was in London browsing through a few shops that sold antiquarian books, I happened upon a little leather-bound job that bore a publication date of 1711. It was appropriately entitled *Herbes for Divers Diseases in Man and Beaste Alike.* Being the son of a bookman myself and obviously deeply interested in medicinal plant lore, I was enthralled with my delightful find.

But I nearly suffered a severe bout of apoplexy when I looked at the price marked inside. The £500 figure in those days translated into an equivalent of $1,500 U.S. It took me a few seconds to catch my breath and recover from such sticker shock. Being the resourceful individual I am, however, I wasn't about to let something like this keep me from gaining access to the information inside.

So, I assumed the "library mode" and found a quiet corner of the bookshop where I could read and copy on note paper those items that interested me the most. I was probably there for a couple of hours and, after returning this very old book to its rightful shelf, left with a number of handwritten pages.

The book, which oddly enough never gave an author, mentioned two herbs in particular as being *exceptional* for the release of stones and the diminishing of the excruciating pain they induce. These were pellitory-of-the-wall *(Parietaria officinalis)* and catnip (always spelled with an "e" in England, as in cat*n*e*p). The first is a common wild plant and the second a popular garden herb found throughout the British Isles.

This is what that ancient volume had to say about the first common weed in the olde English in prevalent use then. "Pellitory of the wall boyled, and the decoction of it drunken, helpeth such as are vexed with an old cough, the gravell and stone, in bothe man and beaste. It is good against the difficultie of making water, and stopping of the same, not onely inwardly, but also outwardly applied upon the region of the bladder, in manner of a fomentation of warme bathing, with spunges or double clouts, or such like."

What's more amazing is that this same remedy still prevails today and is one of the most popular medicines employed by medical herbalists and animal doctors throughout the British Isles. The entire herbe is generally used. One large tablespoon of chopped plant is added to a pint of boiling water, covered, and steeped for 30 minutes before being strained and given to the person or creature suffering from renal calculi. It is best administered when the stomach is empty. Nothing but a fresh batch of this tea should be put in an animal's water dish and more should be added when the other has been drunk.

Pellitory-of-the-wall is nearly impossible to find in America, but may be ordered through a couple of British herbal apothecaries:

Iden Croft Herbs Ltd.
Frittenden Road
Staplehurst
Kent TN12 ODH (England)

A Touch of Spice Ltd.
21 The Highlands
Bexhill-on-Sea
East Sussex TN39 5HL (England)

Fortunately, catnip is quite plentiful on this side of the Atlantic, too. So readers needn't worry about finding a ready supply of it just about everywhere.

This is what I copied from *Herbes for Divers Diseases* . . . in relation to catnip. "The Cats are very much delighted herewith; for the smel of it is so pleasant to them, that they rub themselves upon it, and wallow or tumble about in it, and also feed on the branches and leaves most greedily. . . . It is commended against stones in those thus afflicted, and for stones in Cats and Dogges . . . It is a present helpe for them that be burthen inwardly by meanes of some fall received from an high place, and that are very much bruised and be in much payne. The herbe is to be boyled in wine or mede and given that waye."

The same instructions previously given for the other herb also apply here for catnip. Copious amounts may be consumed in place of regular water with very good success. I must say that I've had hundreds of occasions over the years since reading these words in that rare little book to recommend it without hesitation for kidney stones. It works equally well whether used on humans or animals. I consider catnip to be one of the "miracle herbs" for specific organs such as the kidneys, to keep them in great shape and functioning normally at all times.

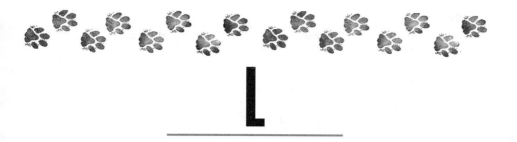

L

LICE

One Woman's Story

First, the good news about cat and dog lice: they won't infest pet owners. And, they're rather uncommon in most household animals.

Now, for the bad news: You'll probably need a magnifying glass of some kind to really look for then, since they're so tiny and go virtually undetected when present.

Ilene Woodruff of Piscataway, New Jersey, shared her own experience with me of lice on her Dalmatian named Suzy. "After I had determined what they were, I decided to give my dog a good shampoo. I used Mane 'n' Tail for this, even though it's supposed to be for horses. But I combined it with a mixture of citrus juices to make it more effective.

"I first took the squeezed juices (one teaspoon each) from a fresh-cut lemon and a lime and blended them in with two table-spoons of the shampoo. I applied this over various parts of Suzy's wet coat and really worked up a good lather, which I left on for about 15 minutes. In the meantime I talked to my dog and distract-ed her long enough to not shake herself nor want to run away.

"Beforehand I had prepared a special rinse consisting of ten drops of tea-tree oil and eight drops of *genuine* turpentine com-bined to a quart of distilled water. The rinse was slow and took longer than usual, because I worked it into every part of her coat. I let that stay on for no more than five minutes. I then gave her a sec-ond and final rinse with cool water, which finished the job.

"All it took was four days of this treatment to *permanently* get rid of all her lice. It did a fantastic job without hurting her."

Litterbox Clumping

How Cat Litter Became an Issue in the First Place

Unless you are a cat owner, you probably would never know about a divisive issue that is generating a mass of public opinion on cat owners as well as veterinarians. Put very simply, it is this: In the past, clay litter was the accepted norm, but now the popular trend is a mixture of clay and sodium bentonite. This makes a more absorbent clay litter that causes the free-flowing mixture to form solid clumps when exposed to moisture. This absorbent property certainly makes the box easier to keep clean. The older plain clay litters were not as finely textured as this newer granular mixtures is, which left detectable urine odors and was harder to deal with.

Consumers have really taken to the improved litter material, thereby greatly increasing its popularity. But clumping litter has one major drawback: It tracks, and the sandlike particles cling to a cat's paw pads. And therein lies the problem that has generated numerous articles both pro and con in relation to the matter.

The Problem from One Perspective

Due to its fine texture, clumping litter comes in contact with a cat's feet, legs, tail, and in the case of male cats, even his genitals, once the animal has urinated or defecated and then covered the waste material over with its hind feet. Later on, when the cat grooms itself, any residual litter on the feline's fur can be accidentally ingested, leaving the cat's digestive system to process and eventually expel it. Besides this, there is the likelihood of clumping litter becoming attractive to both young and older cats if they are suffering from anemia or other illnesses that might induce cravings for clay.

Clumping litter absorbs between 12 to 15 times its weight in liquid and forms a concrete-like solid when wet. This fact has caused great concern with many holistic-minded pet owners who believe that the same cement-like effect happens internally when a cat swallows some of the stuff.

Lisa Newman, a fiercely outspoken critic of clumping cat litter, sees it as a death sentence of sorts for felines everywhere. "I believe it is harmful to animals," she wrote in 1994. "There has been a rise in depressed immune systems, respiratory distress, irritable bowel syndrome, and vomiting (other than hairballs) among cats that I have seen in the past two years. All had one thing in common . . . a clumping product in their litter box. In several cases, simply removing the litter improved the condition of the cat.

"After a period of natural cleansing with herbs . . . cats with 'irritable bowel syndromes' (which had been unsuccessfully treated by veterinarians with a variety of medications) passed copious amounts of a gellike substance. This prompted me to study these clumping litters. I found that when mixed with a small amount of water it maintained its shape, but turned to a gel after repeated contact (60 to 72 hours) or with additional fluid added (as would be found in a cat's digestive tract). One can only imagine what happens when this substance is inhaled. One thing for sure, cats ingest or inhale this substance each time they visit their boxes and when regularly cleaning themselves afterwards."

Furthermore, she insists that even dogs "can be harmed" with this particular litter, since they "love to sneak into the cat box for an (ugh!) treat." Canines doing this "not only ingest the toxins normally found in feline fecal materials, but the coating of clumping litter as well." In her typical straightforward way, she states that owners who love their cats and dogs will use something else other than clumping litter.

Another Opinion on the Matter

Michelle Picozzi of Boulder, Colorado, frequently writes on pet health issues and is a cat lover herself. In a 1997 piece she wrote that the terms "alleged" and "has not been scientifically proven" were used to describe the concerns surrounding clumping litter. She quoted a number of veterinarians, including several who are "holistically oriented," who supported the view that this material isn't harmful to the health of felines.

Other health problems believed to be linked to clumping litter include respiratory failure (on account of the silica dust) and immune depression, brain impairment, and kidney dysfunction (because of the aluminum present). Ms. Picozzi is of the opinion that the evidence against clumping litter is extremely thin and makes for a weak case that it's bad for cats.

Litter Alternatives

To her credit, though, Ms. Picozzi, along with Ms. Newman, have proposed other materials that may work just as well for the litter box and would be a lot safer. A short list of what they include is given here:

Cedar shavings

Citrus peels

Clay (nonclumping)

Corn cobs (ground)

Grain (mixed varieties)

Grass pellets

Newspapers (recycled)

Paper (recycled)

Peanut hulls (ground)

Pine needles

Pine sawdust

Sand/pea gravel mix

Wheat

Wood chips (mixed)

Cat owners should always check to be sure that their litter material "is free of any deodorizers, colors, or drying agents which could be potentially harmful," Ms. Newman noted.

LIVER PROBLEMS

How Pet Livers Get Damaged

In his book, *Dr. Pitcairn's Complete Guide to Natural Health for Dogs & Cats* (Emmaus, PA: Rodale Press, 1995), the author makes this curious observation on page 287: "Liver malfunction is caused by many conditions. Some factors are viral infections or the swallowing of poisonous substances, but in *most cases it's hard to tell just what initiated the problem.*" (I have added italics for emphasis.)

Those of us who are intimately acquainted with what goes into commercial pet foods have no problem discerning where a good majority of liver disorders originate. In their January 1998 newsletter, *Love of Animals,* Dr. Bob Goldstein and his wife, Susan, featured an interesting article entitled, "The Truth About Canned Dog and Cat Foods." They note that many so-called "naturally preserved" pet foods contain meat by-products that usually come "from diseased cows or sick chickens." "These are *terrible foods*" they warn their readers. And the fact that they contain chemical preservatives (to keep the high fat content from going rancid) and artificial coloring agents and dyes (for eye appeal of pet owners), not to mention appetite stimulants (salt, sugar, glucose, sucrose, fructose, phosphoric acid) only makes their impact upon the average animal liver that much more deadly.

The second source for liver problems in animals is the numerous chemical sprays used around the house, in the yard and on pets themselves to keep them free of ticks and fleas. From aerosol deodorants to weed killers, our pets are being constantly exposed to myriad chemicals that gradually build up in their systems and can prove potentially damaging to their livers.

Health Restoration Through Juice Therapy

The best approach to solving a liver dilemma in your cat or dog is to rely upon liquids, since they go fast and easily into the system and can do the best job of healing. Below are two recipes that can be quickly made in a blender. The first recipe is my own creation while the second one belongs to the Goldstein Food Plan for recovering animals and is given here with their kind permission.

CREAM OF CARROT COCKTAIL

1 cup goat's milk (fresh, canned, or packaged)

1 cup carrots, coarsely cut

½ cup sunflower seeds (shelled)

¼ cup walnuts (shelled)

¼ cup almonds (shelled)

¼ teaspoon dandelion powder (the emptied contents from two gelatin capsules of dandelion)

¼ teaspoon milk-thistle-seed extract (the emptied contents of two gelatin capsules of milk-thistle seed)

½ teaspoon beet-root-juice powder*

½ cup spring or purified water

Blend for two minutes until a smooth consistency is formed. Divide into thirds, serve one portion now to the pet in its drinking dish and refrigerate the rest for later feedings.

GOLDSTEIN LIVER COCKTAIL

¼ cup distilled or filtered pure water

½ cup freshly extracted organic carrot juice

½ cup freshly extracted celery juice (high in naturally occurring minerals)

1 tablespoon aloe vera juice

1 tablespoon powdered wheat grass or barley grass* (these super-green foods provide energy)

1 tablespoon nutritional yeast

400 IU vitamin E

In a blender gently mix all ingredients on the lowest speed possible. Only the fresh drink with freshly extracted juices gives you the live enzymes the liver needs in order to totally recuperate. Force-feed animals who are off their feed; however, don't overfeed and cause vomiting. Cats and small and medium dogs can eat two to five tablespoons per day while large and giant breeds can get ten tablespoons.

*Consult the Product Appendix under Pines for obtaining the beet-juice powder and cereal grasses.

LONELINESS

The Social Nature of Creatures

For all of their many differences, humans and animals share at least one common trait: They love company and hate being alone. In the average American town it is quite common to find cats on the loose darting in and out of alleyways in pairs or *several* unfenced dogs roaming a neighborhood together. Deer move in herds, wolves and coyotes run in packs, geese fly in flocks, and fish swim in schools. Throughout much of the animal kingdom, one can always find beasts, birds, and sea creatures that mingle in societies. This is typical behavior, even for the insect kingdom: bees hive, wasps nest, ants colonize, and mosquitoes and gnats swarm together. Scientists who study the social behaviors of such creatures large and small consider such congregating to be the rule rather than the exception.

There are, however, a number of isolated examples that indicate peculiar individuality apart from group functions: the rogue elephant, the lone whale, the single bear, the reclusive mouse, and the solitary fly. For different reasons, each of these life forms has chosen to go it alone separate from its companions. Animal behavior specialists understand some of the reasons for this, but for others they do not. Still, they are agreed upon one point: Creatures of nearly every description and size, like humans, need members of their own kind around quite frequently; otherwise, they tend not to survive very long.

Imposed Isolation

Long ago in the distant past, our earliest ancestors unwittingly created group separations when they took young wolf or tiger cubs from their mothers and raised them for hunting and companionship purposes. Today's many descendants from these first pets are automatically born into isolated circumstances that quickly separate them from their mothers. Puppies and kittens offered for sale by well-intentioned people may look and act cute, but deep inside they still carry the ancient genes of group behavior. At heart they are social creatures of habit and instinct and possess a sense of belonging to someone or something that becomes better defined as they grow older.

In my own life, I raised a German shepherd (Timothy) from puppy to full-grown dog and a mixed Persian-Siamese (Jake) from kitten to feisty tom. I therefore know something myself about these innate emotions that are part of practically every creature. In the beginning, when my life wasn't so busy, I devoted a great deal of time and effort in getting close to each of my pets. But as my reputation in the alternative-health arena grew, so did the demands for my time from many different clients. My extensive traveling left my dog and later my cat without the benefit of the master they had grown to love very much.

Tim started roaming away from home when I lived with my father and brother in the south-central Utah community of Manti. This was totally uncharacteristic of him, but he managed to do it every time I went on another long lecture or research trip somewhere in the world. One time, it was his misfortune to enter a neighbor's chicken coop a few blocks away. The unsympathetic owner obtained what he considered to be just retribution with his hunting rifle for a few dead chickens. My family buried Tim while I was away. Upon returning home and learning the facts, I visited his simple grave site and spent some time there to console my broken heart.

After that I went for several years without another pet. I actually acquired my cat as a present for a staff member, who took care of it in our research center in Salt Lake City. When that individual eventually moved on to other things, the rest of my staff and I were left with a nearly matured cat. Since none of the others were cat lovers, it became my lot in life to take care of Jake.

Over the course of the next several years, we became very much attached to each other. And while it was obvious he missed me when I sometimes traveled, the presence of other office staff kept him fairly secure. But the moment I returned and entered the office, upon hearing my voice he would promptly emerge from wherever he was secreted or resting and race like the wind into our reception room, walking around me with his tail in constant motion and meowing incessantly.

As I reviewed both Tim's wandering and Jake's secluding himself in my absence, I realized that lengthy and frequent separation from the person (myself) they had become deeply attached to eventually led each of my pets toward strange changes not consistent with previous behavioral patterns. The loneliness that such isolation imposed resulted in a gradual breakdown of rational thinking and normal emotions. In a sense, both of their early terminations of life—Jake, too, acted out when we had finally to be separated permanently—were partly my fault for not being around them more often as in former times. From these combined experiences I learned a valuable lesson: *do not get a pet unless you are willing to invest lots of time and emotional energy in establishing a meaningful and lasting relationship.*

Companionship Works Both Ways

Not only do household pets benefit from frequent human contact, but their owners also receive mental and emotional well being. An article entitled "The Healing Power of Pets: A Look at Animal-Assisted Therapy," in the September 1997 issue of *Alternative Therapies* journal, touched on this. The editor, Larry Dossey, M.D., presented compelling evidence to show that cats and dogs can bring a measure of peace and happiness to the lives of the lonely and disturbed. Where psychologists and psychiatrists fail to help, such small animals assist in remarkable ways.

Cats and dogs have incredible intuitive instincts far beyond human capacity. They can discern inner conflict and trouble in their owners of which others may be totally unaware. In their unique ways some of them attempt to bring comfort to bad situations. Dennis Stillings of Waimea, Hawaii, shared the following experiences he had some time ago as evidence of the amazing healing power connected with pet companionships.

"I noticed that the cat of a friend who suffered from a then-undiagnosed severe liver disease would jump up and lie down gently across my friend's liver whenever she reclined on the couch or in bed. She finally consulted a doctor, who discovered the malady and prescribed natural remedies that improved the problem greatly. But the cat was the first one who mysteriously detected it.

"The cat of another friend who suffered from severe depression and migraine would frequently lie down behind my friend's head, like an airline pillow. Mere chance, you say? Perhaps, but who really knows for sure?

"More bizarre, however, is the case of another female friend who suffered from severe vaginitis, which was treated unsuccessfully with cortisone cream. At the same time this disorder arose, my friend obtained a small female dog who promptly developed the same symptoms—to the extent that the animal chewed itself raw in the nether regions.

"Because the cortisone failed to work, my friend consulted with a homeopath, who provided her with a successful remedy. She was cured, but the dog continued to suffer. I suggested that she give the homeopathic medicine to the dog. She complied and the dog totally recovered in just a few days."

Evident Signs of Loneliness

In the best-seller *Dr. Pitcairn's Complete Guide to Natural Health for Dogs & Cats* (Emmaus, PA: Rodale Press, Inc., 1995), the author explains that early in his profession he began making connections between the outward physical manifestations of a pet's health problems with the more hidden emotional distresses. External problems are often symptomatic of "a loss of attention, relationship or territory." The health of a pet, in fact, can be greatly affected "by recurrent feelings" of loneliness, rejection, depression, anxiety, anger, and tension.

Although cats and dogs each express their own frustrations in different ways, there are enough shared similarities to pinpoint something wrong in their psyches. I've compiled a short list of the most common features to look for as an indication of animal loneliness, depression, or feelings of rejection.

1. *Intense Scratching.* If a small animal is continually scratching itself and the probable cause are *not* fleas or other insects, food or chemical allergies, or environment-related, then rest assured it's most likely emotional in nature.

2. *Extreme Restlessness.* Tail chasing, excessive licking, and fidgetiness are frequently seen in animals lacking attention and emotional care.

3. *Frequent Urination.* One of the sure signs of an unloved or infrequently loved pet is for it to discharge the contents of its bladder at random. Sometimes, when this isn't enough, an adult animal will resort to unexpected defecation in the most inappropriate areas imaginable. It's the pet's way of voicing extreme dissatisfaction with an owner's apparent neglect and saying, as it were, "Hey, master (or mistress) . . . better start showing some attention this way or be prepared for some R-E-A-L-L-Y B-I-G action on my part!"

4. *Property Destruction.* This is the final, all-out assault on an insensitive and selfish owner. In the mind of the emotionally stressed pet, it has become the "big enchilada" of last resorts. An unloved animal will remember what are its owner's favorite pieces of furniture or clothing and go after those objects with a vengeance peculiar only to dogs and cats. An expensive chair may get chewed on, a fine wood desk scratched to hell, or a blouse, shirt, or pants shredded to ribbons. The attitude by now is, "What have I got to lose? Either love me, dammit, or else send me away to someone who can."

Coping with Animal Stress

Upon seeing such ill-mannered or unanticipated behavior from their otherwise "normal" animals, the initial reaction of many pet owners is to haul them off to the local veterinary clinic for the human equivalent of Valium or some other equally strong medication to calm them down. Thus doped up, the animals become seemingly docile. But this passivism is only temporary and unless corrected in other ways, will require further drug therapy.

The real key to controlling a distraught pet, Dr. Pitcairn noted in his book, lies with its owner. "The owner's attitudes . . . about the . . . disturbance can have a pronounced effect on the outcome." Inappropriate pet behaviors "often mirror those of the primary person with whom the [animals] are bonded." "By paying special attention to emotional issues in the home, it's possible to foster the kind of positive emotional climate that helps a pet maximize its ability to restore and maintain health.

Dealing with Dogs

Pets, more than children, as a rule, are capable of soaking up positive or negative emotions from those whom they've grown especially attached to. Barbara Woodhouse of Great Britain, who has trained more than 17,000 dogs in her lifetime, believes that abundant love and measured firmness are paramount to winning over an animal. In her book *No Bad Dogs* (New York: Summit Books, 1982), she makes the following important observations.

"I think . . . love is of paramount importance, and I constantly hug, kiss and play joyfully with my pupils even if I have had to be extremely firm with them to achieve initial obedience. The result is that there enters the dog's mind a memory of affection and fun rather than fear of correction. . . . Dogs don't object to fair correction. In fact . . . the most loving dogs often seem to belong to owners to whom I would hate to be related in any way.

"In a dog's mind, a master or a mistress to love, honor and obey is an absolute necessity. The love is dormant in the dog until brought into full bloom by an understanding owner. Thousands of dogs *appear* to love their owners . . . with enthusiastic wagging of the tail and jumping up [and following] them about their houses happily. To the normal person seeing [this], the affection [seems] true and deep. But to the experienced dog trainer this outward show isn't enough. The true test of *real* love takes place when the dog has got the opportunity to go out on its own as soon as a door is left open by mistake and it goes off and often doesn't return for hours. The dog loves only its home comforts and the attention it gets from its family; it doesn't truly love the master or mistress as they fondly think. *True* love in dogs is apparent when a door is left open and the dog still stays happily within earshot of its owner. For the owner must be the be-all and end-all of a dog's life.

"To achieve this the owner has to master the dog at the same time or other as the leader of the pack did in bygone days. There must be no question as to who is the boss of the house; it must be the owner.

Dogs not only love owners who have had at one time a battle of wills for supremacy; they adore them, for a dog is *really* a subservient creature by nature, longing to trust his true love to someone's heart.

"Giving praise and affection is where a multitude of owners fail their dogs. A pat and a kind word are not enough in the initial training of dogs; the atmosphere must be charged with a certain excitement, for dogs are very sensitive to excitement. When they have done right, they love having the wildest show of affection and a good romp. Dull owners make dull dogs. . . .

"Dogs love laughter, clapping and jokes . . . Try smiling at everyone you meet down the street; you will be amazed how many complete strangers smile back before they zip up again, realizing they don't know you. It is the same with dogs even if they don't know you; they respond with a smile and a clap if they have done well. *They watch your eyes and face for the happy sign that you are pleased.* I am intensely sorry for the dogs who see no smiles on their owners' faces. You can't train a dog well if you are unhappy; your tenseness communicates itself to the dog, and the dog becomes depressed.

"People should understand life from a dog's point of view before blaming him for everything that goes wrong. Mothers-to-be buy every book they can on baby welfare, but hundreds of people buy dogs with very little knowledge of them and then blame the dog for behavior they don't approve of." Ms. Woodhouse then suggests that before anyone buys or obtains a dog, he or she should inquire about the animal or read up on the breed being considered to see if it may be right for that individual. Mismatchings are frequently the underlying cause to loneliness in dogs: Happy dogs are those that have been paired to firm but kindly personalities who will treat them well all their lives.

Ms. Woodhouse's most sage admonition for achieving mental and emotional well-being in your canine is this: "Remember, 'dog' spelled backward is 'god,' and you should be 'god' to your dog!"

Conforming to Cats

Cats, on the other hand, are of an entirely different stripe. They are highly individualistic and, more often than not (as every cat owner should know) have minds of their own. "They do whatever they damn well please when it suits their particular fancy and pleasure!" one long-time expert and judge at numerous cat shows told me awhile back. In his opinion, "cats have only three things on their minds: themselves, mice, and sleep!"

I can't vouch for the psychological accuracy of this statement, but I can say from personal experience with Jake, my former Persian-Siamese mix, that while he "accommodated" me to some extent, I largely "conformed" to his ways of doing things. And it is this "conforming" on the part of a cat owner that makes for a healthy and happy animal relationship.

Some years ago I attended a lecture given by the internationally renowned German animal trainer Gunther Gebel-Williams of circus fame. He had spent almost 45 years handling big cats under the Big Top. He mentioned that he regularly kept large and powerful Bengal and Siberian tigers as house pets. And handled them, not with the customary whip-and-chair method, but by talking to them. "The more you verbally communicate with your cats, the closer you and they become," he said. "Cats know if you are going to be nice to them by the tone of your voice, not the words that you speak."

Gunther firmly believed that cats, more than other animals, had evolved over time with an innate sense of ESP (extra-sensory perception). This nonverbal language permits them to sort out situations in their minds long before we humans can. And this nonverbal skill isn't just limited by time or space. An intuitive owner can communicate with his or her cat while sitting in a chair on the couch some distance away. Gunther shared with his audience how he learned to pick up the feelings of occasional loneliness in some of his huge house pets by "listening with the soul" rather than the ear.

"Learning how to communicate with your cat is pretty much a two-way street," he informed his audience. "It's give and take on both ends: command and listen on your part; consider and act on the cat's end. Then it may go in the other direction: think and send, for you to receive and conform." This doesn't necessarily mean that your cat always gets the upper hand (or claw) in things, but that specific boundaries of authority acceptable to both parties are established and mutually adhered to.

"If you treat your cat with *love,* if you treat your cat with *respect,* if you treat your cat as an *intelligent* and thinking animal capable of making wise decisions, then your cat will respond in many ways that will simply astonish you," Gunther declared. "The secret to a heavenly relationship with the feline species," he added with a grin, "is to let your cat know you are its master, but also *never* to forget that she is *your* mistress!"

Gunther told us that cats transmit more external signals with regard to their internal feelings and dispositions than any other animals he knows of. "*Watch their body language* at all times!" he insisted. Eyes wide open mean kitty is awake and raring to go. A glint, however, may indicate some mischief in mind, so be prepared for that. Cats need to be outdoors enough to vent their built-up physical energies from periods of confinement. Cats, by nature, contain an innate, genetic urge to flee from danger or hurtle at top speed after prey. That is why they need to be let outside every so often to relieve themselves by suddenly "exploding" into frenetic bursts of high-voltage energy and madly dashing about for no apparent reason. Otherwise, they're apt to do it inside, where considerable damage can be done to household furnishings, especially if those cats are as large as Gunther's kitties!

The mouth is another area to watch. It does more than meow or roar. When kitty is relaxed, its mouth and lips are in normal position. But, if open and slightly curled, be on your guard; this is to be taken seriously.

A cat's ears are extremely sensitive and acutely attuned to a wide range of sounds. They are also wonderful barometers of a cat's mood. Gunther claimed he could tell more about his big cats' moods by how they positioned their ears than by looking into their eyes, as many cat owners are apt to do.

Relaxed but alert ears move calmly but determinedly around an area, gauging sound, direction, and meaning. A cat given plenty of attention and attached to its owner will generally have it ears lie this way. But submissive or fearful ears are usually pulled back, lying against the head. They let the owner know that kitty isn't happy and is feeling anxiety about something. A wise owner will gently stroke or brush its fur while speaking in soft tones to it to help allay this apparent stress. Aggressive ears are indicated by a slight rotation. The ear is in its normal position, but faces forward. The ear looks like the wings of an airplane, ready for fight or flight. Only some emotional mixture will induce a cat to make its ears twitch. Sometimes this can indicate great joy, but more often than not it usually means fear or aggression.

But Gebel-Williams's favorite part of a cat's anatomy is its tail. "This forms the most beautiful speech on earth. That tail conveys more information about how he or she is feeling than any other part," he said. Waving tails in felines generally convey just the opposite meaning that wagging tails in friendly canines do. Many an unfortunate person has been badly mauled because that individual mistook a cat's wagging tail as a sign of friendship. Relaxed tails mean kitty is at peace with itself and the world around it.

After returning home from a long circus tour, Gunther would usually be met by his huge tigers holding their tails directly vertical while displaying quivering body motions. This was their excited way of "welcoming me back again," he stated.

A swishing tail is something to be on the lookout for. In the side thumping, window-wiper mode, "kitty is really pissed off at something and needs space and to be left alone for awhile." It's just the opposite of happy, tail-wagging dogs.

Inquisitive tails are especially fun to watch. Curious cats will often conduct their own fascinating treasure hunts, prancing around with their tails pointed straight up. Some cats, though, are fond of adding an enchanting little curlicue to the tip of their tails for good measure. The delight of discovery is often manifested in such upwardly pointed, but end-moving tail motions. They signal a wonderful mixture of curiosity, excitement, and fun.

Your Pet Is What You Are

In the last decade considerable research advances have been made in the mind-body connection relative to human health. Scientists worldwide now understand that the way we feel mentally and emotionally largely determines how we will be physically. Wherefore, more and more doctors are considering the thoughts of the mind and emotions of the heart as playing pivotal roles in the initiation, progression, and final outcome of many organic diseases.

Only recently, though, have a few practitioners of veterinary medicine begun applying the same logic toward sick animals. And the lack of or loss of existing love and attention is turning out to be responsible for a rising number of common animal health problems mentioned earlier in the text. As Dr. Pitcairn correctly points out in his book: "Pets often seem to soak up angry, sad or fearful feelings from family members who are experiencing tension or conflict over issues that have nothing to do with the animal."

The animal is inclined to think it is to blame for such negative hostilities, when, in fact, it isn't. But trying to convince the animal such isn't the case at all is easier said than done. Only by being relaxed and at peace themselves, can loving owners impart a similar sense of well-being to those animals they care very much about. Under such glad circumstances, pets seem to thrive and do exceptionally well.

LYME DISEASE

A Problem that Really Ticks off Pet Owners

Ticks are ugly little buggers that can make a person's or animal's life sheer hell. These dreadful but exceedingly clever little critters not only can make your skin crawl with fear, but they move about on the skin's surface looking for a nice "bed-and-breakfast" to burrow down into and snack in for a while. They are in tiny form the equivalent of welfare queens, drug addicts, alcoholics, drunk drivers, child abusers, bigots, rapists, murderers, spies, politicians, thugs, religious con men, and other types of human parasites who prey on society.

Before Count Dracula there were ticks, the ultimate bloodsuckers of the insect world. They get into animals and people by special built-in heat sensors that suddenly announce in tick language, "Get ready, fellows—lunch is coming!" They then drop off the undersides of leaves and twigs where they've been napping and land (without parachute) on the unlucky passersby. In less than an hour they will dine in style.

I remember many years ago trekking with some archaeologists through the heart of the Guatemalan jungle. It was as hot as a furnace and the stifling air made me think of Dante's *Inferno*. The ticks our group encountered were super-sized in comparison to regular ticks (but still small, mind you). Every evening the same ritual was performed over and over again by each of us, one on the other: We held a lit cigarette close enough to the skin (without actually burning it) until those little creeps backed out where we could then properly dispense with them.

Ticks are a nuisance no matter where you travel on this globe; they're just part of this "fallen world" (as opposed to Conan Doyle's *Lost World*). While humans can do something about getting them out, animals can't without some assistance from us. The longer they remain in man or beast, the greater the risk of contracting Lyme disease. Medical authorities claim that an infected tick must gorge itself nonstop on blood for about 13 hours before it can leave its disease-causing bacterial calling card.

Until only recently there wasn't much a person could do to rid himself or his pet of ticks. Old standbys such as smoldering matches or applications with Vaseline, hog lard, alcohol, or solvent weren't that practical. Nor was the use of tweezers—most common method. In fact, if the truth were known, that way probably *increases* the risk of injecting Lyme disease into the bloodstream. Regular tweezers, while putting out the tick's behind, generally left the head intact.

But now a revolutionary new device from Scandinavia enables the entire insect to be removed. This easy-to-use, cylindrical, surgical-steel device reverses the burrowing action of the tick, so that the tiny devil can be taken out in a more efficient way. (See Product Appendix under Scandinavian Naturals for more information.)

Supplements to Use

Getting high-powered botanicals and nutrients into the affected animal is of prime importance. I've found that the following items work particularly well in fighting the fever and inflammation that traditionally accompany this insidious infection:

- *Liquid Japanese aged-garlic extract*—20 drops in the back of the throat every three hours (use less for cats and small dogs)

- *Echinacea and goldenseal-root combination*—two capsules daily for small and twice that amount for large pets

- *Yucca-fluid extract*—12 drops morning and evening; double that for big animals

- *Liquid vitamin C*—one-half teaspoon for cats and small canines to one tablespoon for big pets, twice daily on both

- *Red-clover tea*—Give in place of water. Steep one-half cup in one pint spring or distilled water (no tap water, please), covered, for 20 minutes. Strain and use when cool.

(*Note:* See Product Appendix under Wakunaga for garlic; Holistic Animal Care for the other herbs; and your local health-food store for the vitamin C and red-clover blossoms.) (Also see Infection and Ticks for more information.)

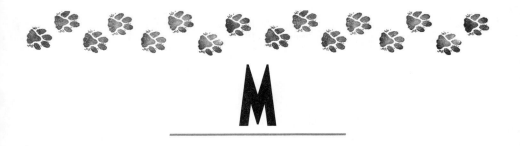

M

MANGE

An Australian Solution

Jackie Fitzgerald is a successful practicing herbalist in the land "down under." She believes in and regularly uses many homeopathic preparations as well in her practice—something I personally don't believe in. But I respect her for her skill and knowledge in the healing arts. (I don't believe in homeopathy because I feel it is an art inspired from dark sources. An herbalist is one who uses herbs in their entirety and not fractioned portions of them. A homeopath, on the other hand, uses extracted parts of herbs in combination with non-plant agents, some of which are deadly poisons, i.e., black widow spider, cobra venom, arsenic, lead, etc.)

A few years ago, she wrote this: "A very effective treatment for mange can be made by giving whole (minced) garlic and by making a lotion of garlic and rubbing it on the animal's body every day. Simply mince up 30–40 cloves of garlic and place them in a gallon container. Pour boiling spring water over the garlic and keep the container covered to prevent the evaporation of the essential oils. Use as a lotion by rubbing on to the animal daily. Continue this treatment until the condition is cleared up. And, as with all herbal usage, don't forget to use some common sense."

(Also see under Itching, Mites, and Skin Problems for additional information.)

MITES

A Proven Mite Buster

Raquel S. from Yorba Linda, California, has found the "perfect solution" (as she calls it) for getting rid of those tiny, annoying pests that invade pets' ears and cause them to scratch incessantly.

"I shampoo the heads, ears, and tails of my golden retriever *and* my Persian once a week," she told me. Then, with a laugh, she added, "Of course Fluffy—that's my cat—fights it all the time, but she knows resisting won't do her any good."

Following this procedure, this female movie-stunt woman dilutes three drops each of yellow-dock and golden-seal tincture in one-and-a-half tablespoons of distilled or filtered water. "I usually put one-half dropperful in each ear canal and gently massage it afterwards. I let my pets shake their heads after doing this, then I blot the openings with several cotton swabs. I administer this treatment once every three days for up to a month. It really helps to get rid of mites in those difficult-to-reach places like the ears."

She also sprays some of this same liquid herbal mixture on the heads and tails of her pets and then lightly rubs it in with her fingers. She informed me on the day we spoke by phone recently that "I had tried some other things recommended by my local veterinarian, but they didn't seem to do the job as effectively as the herbs did." Besides this, she added, "I prefer using things on my pets that are more natural and safe for them. I believe it's morally wrong to use anything on your animals that isn't natural to begin with." (See Product Appendix under Nature's Answer for obtaining these tinctures.) (See also Mange.)

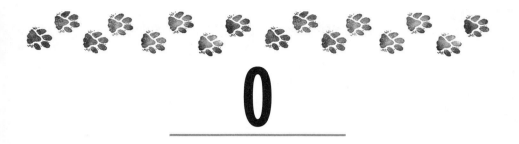

0

OBESITY

Cat and Owner Stay Slim

Duane King works on Wall Street as a part-time stockbroker. He lives alone with his five-year-old male tabby Stirling in "a decent flat" (as he likes to call it). He also likes to run a lot and is quite good at it, as a matter of fact. He missed by a mere 13 seconds of setting a new record in the New York Marathon in 1996.

"Well, I lost a marathon," he said whimsically, "but, at least, I manage to keep my cat slim." Just then Stirling walked by and rubbed himself against his owner's leg. Duane hefted the cat up and handed it to me for inspection. "There's not an ounce or inch of fat anywhere on that bod," he said with jubilation.

As I put Stirling on my lap and carefully examined him, he continued purring contentedly. Duane was right: There was no appearance of obesity, no thick waist, no dandruff or oiliness, and no unpleasant smell. In fact, this looked like one very healthy cat!

So, I wanted to know after putting Stirling down to the floor, "How do you keep your pet so slender, when cats this age and older are notorious for becoming fat?"

Duane then slowly began to recite for me the program he developed early on when his cat was still a kitten "to keep him slender for all of his nine lives," he said with a chuckle. With each meal, he adds the following items, and has been doing so for about four years:

> 1 teaspoon of minced fish mix (mackerel, salmon, and sardines) for their coenzyme Q10 contents

1 teaspoon finely grated *raw* vegetable mix (equal parts carrot and celery)

3 tablespoons mineral water

⅛ teaspoon vitamin C powder (about 325 mg.)

½ teaspoon vitamin E oil*

*The author recommends using Rex Wheat Germ Oil. (See the Product Appendix under Anthropological Research Center for more information.)

Duane then explained the logic behind each of his singular choices. "Coenzyme Q10 and vitamins C and E seem to keep the metabolic functions always high enough so excess fat is always burned off and never stored. The vegetable fiber and mineral water keep his bowels pretty regular." Duane also mentioned that "maybe two or three times a week I'll mince a garlic clove and include it with both daily feedings."

"One thing that I try and do a *lot* of that other cat owners may not take the time to do," he added, "is to show Stirling l-o-v-e! I'll kiss him on the nose or forehead, pet him quite a bit, hug him often, and play with him a great deal. This I do instead of giving him cat snacks, which would only make him fat as a butterball anyway.

"I also set aside plenty of rec[reation] time for both of us. I use rubber balls, yarn balls, and anything else he might find intriguing enough to play or romp around with. I see that he gets adequate exercise every day, just like his owner." With that statement, Duane then patted his abdomen hard to show it was as solid as brick. "No love handles here," he added reassuringly.

How to Help Your Dog Lose Weight

Dr. Bob and Susan Goldstein of Westport, Connecticut, are world-famous experts on natural animal care. He owns and operates the Northern Skies Veterinary Center and she is an avid writer and pet nutrition authority. I read their *Love of Animals* newsletter periodically.

Bob and Susan tackled the issue of animal obesity in their October 1995 newsletter (see Appendix II for subscription information) and gave permission for extensive excerpting therefrom.

Although their advice pertains mostly to canines, some of it is equally applicable to felines.

They have what they like to call "The Monday 1-Minute Weight Checkup" that you should always conduct with your pet. "Just as animals have their unique personalities, they also have unique metabolic rates. The issue of determining obesity in dogs and cats is a simple one. All you need to do is tune into your animal and do what [we] do at home with [our] 'kids.'

Every Monday, [we] place Annie on a table that's waist-high. (For large dogs like our Boxer, Jack, you can come down to their level.) [We] palpate along Annie's ribs. There should be a nice firm layer of skin covering the ribs. (If you can't feel the ribs at all, that tells you something right there.) Then [Susan or I] travel to the soft spot just behind the last rib and stop. If [either of us] feels a soft pouch of fatty tissue there, then [we] know that [we] need to adjust Annie's food and exercise, and maybe lengthen the time of her meal-skip."

They warn against using commercial foods prescribed by veterinarians that are specifically intended for animal weight loss. "These diets are often loaded with indigestible fillers (empty calories) that will take weight off. The problem is, after weeks or months eating this nutritionally void food, the animal will become ravenous, causing weight gain. Once again, conventional medicine is treating obesity as a symptom to be stamped out—even if it means starving your pet [to do so]."

They then provide readers with what is described as "The Easiest Diet *You've* Even Been On." "Start with the basics," they insist, "so you can see results in a month's time."

- *Reduce commercial food* intake by one third. Continue feeding the same amount of fresh raw vegetables, the same dollops of low-fat yogurt and the olive oil. [See Fatigue and the subsection, "Super-Charged Meals for Pooped-Out Pets."] The extra fiber in the veggies will help stave off hunger pangs. The yogurt aids digestion and the olive oil is so digestible that it's just fine to keep this type of fat in the diet.

- *Increase exercise by tacking 10 minutes onto your daily dog walks or buying some new cat toys.* [We] think the Cat Dancer and the Kitty Fishing Reel are the best. Rotate toys, so periodically there's something else new for your cat.

- *Switch to 'lite' or senior food* if your animal is older or has a chronic weight problem. Mix the new food in gradually increasing proportions to the current food. Start with 5% new food to 95% old. Bob and I have had success with Natural Life, Cornucopia and Lick Your Chops formulations.

- *Feed healthy snacks and treats:* carrots, low-fat popcorn, shredded wheat, melon (which cats love), brown rice cakes and chunks of organic apples. These high-fiber, low-fat snacks will ease hunger pangs and the psychological need for treats.

- *Meal-skip once a week.* A 12-hour weekly fast improves the health status of every animal over a year old. Do not fast sick animals unless under the supervision of a holistic veterinarian.

The Goldsteins then offer "secret weapons" that help to "melt the pounds" away. They refer to these as their "fat-busting supplements." "You can restore your dog's or cat's health—even if you think losing weight is a lost cause. This special combination of foods and vitamins gears up your animal's metabolism and breaks down fat.

"The seaweed kelp is a natural source of iodine, which can increase metabolism of a sluggish thyroid. You can buy kelp at health food stores. [We've] included vitamin B-6, because, like the kelp, it aids the metabolism. Many pharmacies carry the individual B vitamins in 25 mg. tablets. For smaller animals, you can cut a 25 mg. tablet in half.

"Lecithin breaks down fats, helping the body to eliminate them. Buy the capsules at a health food store. Apple cider vinegar added to the drinking water will also help to dissolve fats. Please do not give your dog or cat vinegar unless it's organic.

"These dosages are adequate for approximately every 25 lbs. of body weight. Cut in half for most cats and increase accordingly for larger dogs. You do not have to be exact. Once your animal establishes a healthy weight, you can discontinue the fat-busters or use them one week on, one week off."

GOLDSTEINS' FAT-BUSTING SUPPLEMENTS

Kelp—1 teaspoon sprinkled on food, A.M. and P.M.
Lecithin—1 capsule 2 times daily
Vitamin B-6—25 mg. daily
Organic apple-cider vinegar—1 teaspoon in drinking water 2 times daily

GOLDSTEINS' FAT-BUSTING DIET

(PORTIONS ARE FOR 25-POUND ANIMAL; ADJUST ACCORDINGLY)

3 ounces lightly steamed skinless chicken
1 cup cooked brown rice
½ cup steamed or raw vegetables, finely chopped
2 teaspoons low-fat yogurt
2 teaspoons extra-virgin olive oil

"[We] are anxious for you to enjoy a slimmer, more energetic, healthier companion. Of course, you don't have to do everything we recommend. One or two steps may trim off a few unneeded pounds. If you know you've got a tough case on your hands, [we encourage] you to try [our] fat busters. [Come] the New Year, you will see dramatic results!" Last, they encourage owners to take before-and-after pictures so that they can see where their pets started and where they eventually ended.

Fasting for Your Pet

Again, we are indebted to the Goldsteins for their medical expertise and nutritional wisdom in giving a sense of proper direction for owners who wish to help their pets lose weight. Fasting has long been a part of true weight loss. Not only is there spiritual significance connected with it for the human experience, but on an animal level it does health wonders.

Bob and Susan explain in their own words. "Meal-skipping can be surprisingly therapeutic for dogs and cats. Fasting your animal frees up energy (normally reserved for digestion) for the body to cleanse itself. It's terrific for pets with joint, intestinal, lung or skin problems. Try skipping a meal weekly, providing a 24 hour fast. Prior to the mini-fast, we like to feed our animals a light meal. Oatmeal, yogurt, and apples, or brown rice, carrots, and olive oil are good choices in place of dog food. These light, low-protein meals are easy to assimilate, setting up the digestive system for rest. On the morning following the fast, feed as usual."

They, however, issue a cautionary note to owners attempting to do this. "If your animal begs for food, offer a carrot, apple or fresh vegetable juice (never tomato or citrus). Do not skip meals for puppies or kittens in the first year; pregnant or nursing mothers; diabetic animals or those with a chronic degenerative disease (without the supervision of a veterinarian); or elderly animals that are experiencing unexplained weight loss (unless under the guidance of a veterinarian)."

They then offer two "Preludes to a Fast":

RECIPE I

"This light meal makes few demands on the digestive system, allowing energy that would normally be expended for digestion to be used for healing."

¼ cup applesauce, organic
1 tablespoon bee pollen
1 cup oatmeal, cooked

Combine ingredients and serve.

CATS AND SMALL DOGS (UP TO 25 POUNDS)	DOGS (50 POUNDS)
½ cup	*1 ½ cups*

RECIPE II

"A higher protein version for animals who become too hungry on the lighter meal."

¼ cup oatmeal, cooked
1 egg yolk, raw
1 teaspoon yogurt
1 tablespoon bee pollen
¼ cup natural commercial food (dry)

(continued)

Place the oatmeal in a bowl. Separately, combine the egg yolk, yogurt, and bee pollen. Mix the oatmeal with the commercial food and add the egg-yogurt mixture.

CATS AND SMALL DOGS (UP TO 25 POUNDS)	DOGS (50 POUNDS)
½ cup	1 ½ cups

Finally, Bob and Susan offer some advice and meal tips for breaking a pet's fast. "Use your intuition as to whether your newly rejuvenated friend prefers veggies or fruits upon completing a fast. If your dog or cat needs the quick energy boost, break the fast with a banana or bite-sized pieces of apple mixed with oatmeal. If you feel that he or she is basically content, the sugar from the fruits may not be necessary. This meal is high in digestible complex carbohydrates and soluble fiber but light enough not to overwhelm the system. By the way, dogs, cats and birds all love peas. We like Tree of Life frozen organic peas."

BREAK-THE-FAST MORNING MEAL

3 carrots, grated

1 handful of last night's leftover peas

2 tablespoons virgin olive oil

3–4 cups oatmeal, cooked

Mix the grated carrots, peas, and olive oil with the oatmeal and serve.

CATS AND SMALL DOGS (UP TO 25 POUNDS)	DOGS (50 POUNDS)
½ to 1 cup	2 cups

(The preceding information was used with permission of the Goldsteins and comes from their booklet, *Super Foods and Healing Meals for Pets,* which was a free giveaway when pet owners subscribed to their monthly newsletter. I am grateful for their generosity in letting me use this material here.)

Shedding Pounds During the Dog Days of Summer

In their July 1996 issue of *Love of Animals,* Susan Goldstein puts some more of her nutritional knowledge to work to come up with some innovative ways to help your pets keep off the weight during the long, hot summer months.

"In [the] summer[time], I not only use the water [that my] asparagus is steamed in for my animals but [I] also share full stalks with them. . . . Introducing this green broth is one of the simplest ways you can help your animal lose weight [during the] summer.

"This nutritious broth is a powerful diuretic that energizes older animals who may be retaining water. Plus, the high concentration of chlorophyll purifies the blood and intestines. The elimination of excess fluid cleanses the body of toxins and wastes. Serve asparagus broth only when you plan to be home with your animal for the next four hours because you'll need to escort your buddy outdoors frequently. For cats, of course, leave free access to the litter box.

"If you're gung ho and don't mind a little cooking in the summertime, here's a fun, healthy recipe that will help your animal shed [those summer] pounds."

CHICKEN À LA CANINE (AND FELINE)

"This meal tastes so good that your animal will never suspect he's on a diet. You can feed this meal to dogs as long as you need to in order to take the weight off. For cats, I recommend blending the cooked food in a food processor for better palatability. You can feed this menu to your cat for up to a month. After that time, mix with a commercial base food to ensure that he or she is getting sufficient protein from the diet."

1 cup uncooked brown rice (organic if possible)

2½ cups spring or distilled water

3 ounces chicken (preferably antibiotic-free)

½ cup asparagus, cucumber, or carrots, chopped

2 teaspoons plain low-fat yogurt (organic)

2 teaspoons [extra-]virgin olive oil (optional)

(continued)

Cook rice in water for 20 minutes. Add chopped, boneless, skinless chicken and vegetables and cook another 25 minutes or until all [the] water is absorbed. Add the yogurt and oil. Stir well. Makes 3½ cups.

SERVING AMOUNTS

½ cup for a cat and small dog
1 cup for medium dogs (15–35 pounds)
2 cups for large dogs (50–85 pounds)
2½ to 3½ cups for giant dogs (85+ pounds)

Susan believes in fasting her pets during the summer months. "I have traditionally fasted [them] on Sunday evenings. Most people are amazed when they are greeted the next morning by an enthusiastic, happy dog or cat. I like fasting my animals in the summer because I can add vegetable or fruit juices (fresh carrot, cucumber or melon juice) to [their] water bowl if I feel that some nutrients are needed. I always tune into their actions when my animals fast and I'd like [for] you to do the same [with] yours. [But] do not fast kittens and puppies, and do not fast animals who are sickly or wasting away unless under the supervision of a veterinarian!"

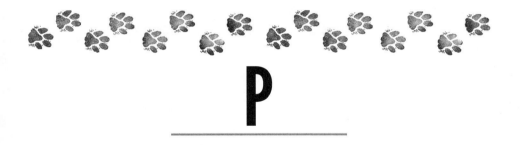

P

PAIN

A Surprising Find

In the preparation of this work, I looked through a number of other books dealing exclusively with the health problems of pets in order to get a better feel for what was out there. One day recently, I consulted about a dozen of them to see what the various authors had to say about the subject of pain.

Imagine my great surprise when I found that over half of these works didn't have anything on pain, nor did they even mention the topic in their indexes. Even a best-seller and oft-consulted reference such as *Dr. Pitcairn's Complete Guide to Natural Health for Dogs & Cats* had nothing listed in the back on "pain" per se. Two well-used emergency references by Bruce Fogle, DVM—*First Aid for Dogs* and *First Aid for Cats* (New York: Penguin Books, 1997)—have only a single entry each for "painkillers" and what to do if a dog or cat were accidentally *poisoned* by something such as aspirin or ibuprofen. Otherwise, nothing else is given on the matter.

More discouraging is the fact that two of the most important reference works in veterinary practice failed to adequately address the issue. *Current Veterinary Therapy X: Small Animal Practice* (Philadelphia: W. B. Saunders Co., 1989), edited by Robert W. Kirk, DVM, has a mere three sentences on what should be done for "Pain Control in Poisoning" situations. The real kicker, though, is the total lack of material dealing with any kind of pain in *The 5 Minute Veterinary Consult: Canine and Feline* (Baltimore: Williams & Wilkins, 1997) written by veterinarians Larry P. Tilley and Francis S.K. Smith, Jr.

Some Light at the End of the Tunnel

Only in a book by Anitra Frazier, entitled *The New Natural Cat: A Complete Guide for Finicky Owners* (New York: Penguin Books, 1990), is there a specific section for pain in the general index, which gives references on seven different pages. Ah, I thought to myself, there is a little light at the end of this dismal tunnel after all. This nationally recognized authority on feline nutrition, grooming, and behavior patterns actually had some worthwhile information on pain control.

Ms. Frazier's favorite nutrient is the mineral calcium. "Calcium calms nerves and raises the threshold for pain and stress," she wrote. She advises cat owners with felines in pain to have their veterinarians "prescribe more calcium" to relieve the excruciating agony. But "to absorb calcium the body needs vitamin D," she adds.

Elsewhere in the text she provides her own nutritional mix for small-animal pain relief:

FRAZIER'S PAIN FORMULA MIX

1 ½ cups brewer's yeast
¼ cup kelp powder
1 cup lecithin granules
2 cups wheat bran
2 cups bone meal

After everything is mixed and put into a plastic covered container, it should be refrigerated. Ms. Frazier suggests adding 2 teaspoons of this mix to a cat's meal per day.

Furthermore, she suggests reducing the sodium content of a feline's diet, since sodium appears to *enhance* pain transmission. I know from personal experience that when humans in great pain are placed on a sodium-restricted diet, the intensity of their pain subsides accordingly. Ms. Frazier recommends, too, that "one-quarter teaspoon bone meal and one droppersful of cod liver oil" be added to the cat's food to provide muscle relaxation and relief from nerve pain.

How One Dog Owner Obtained Relief for His Pet

A business executive in Chicago by the name of Jack owns a pure-bred Labrador. One time a burglar attempted to gain access to the man's nicely furnished house in a posh neighborhood. His faithful dog charged the thief after hearing the sound of broken glass and a window sliding up. The animal grabbed the criminal's leg that was already hanging inside over the sill and started pulling hard on it. The man fell inward hitting the floor pretty hard. The burglar finally managed to get up and with his good leg gave the dog a strong, swift kick to the ribs. The poor animal loosened his hold and gave a loud yelp of pain, which allowed the burglar just enough time to make a hasty retreat from the premises.

When the businessman came home later in the afternoon, he discovered the broken window and his faithful friend lying on the carpet some distance away. Realizing the dog might be seriously hurt, he rushed him off to the veterinary clinic where doctors took X-rays to determine the extent of the injuries. They found no broken bones, just some very badly bruised ribs and muscles. They gave the owner medication to help relieve his pet's suffering and discharged it.

Believing that a nutritional approach was a better answer to drug therapy, Jack consulted with a female co-worker who was into health foods and the like. She, in turn, mentioned to him my *Encyclopedia of Nature's Vitamins and Minerals* (Paramus, NJ: Prentice Hall, 1998) that had just been released a short time before this incident occurred. He borrowed her copy and read in the Product Appendix about two nutritional supplements from Trace Minerals Research of Ogden, Utah. These were Arth-X Plus and Calcium-Magnesium. He found my phone number in the back of the book and gave me a call one morning to see if it would be safe to give some of these tablets to his injured Lab. I told him I didn't think there would be any harm in doing so, but to keep me informed of any unusual developments.

He purchased a bottle of each product from a health food store. He crushed two tablets of each on a cutting board with the bottom of a heavy cast-iron skillet. He then added the powder of these four tablets to his dog's chow *twice daily*. Within a week his beautiful animal showed no further evidence of discomfort and appeared to be pain-free. Jack called again and thanked me for the information, but asked that his privacy be respected when I raised the matter of using his story in this book. That is why his name shall remain anonymous, although the experience is factual. (See Product Appendix under Trace Research for more data on these products.)

The Most Unusual Pain Remedy for Pets I've Ever Heard

As most of us probably know, "life is wonderful," but full of big and little surprises that can sometimes grab and astonish us without advance notice. During the first part of 1998 I was reading the February issue of *Chile Pepper* magazine, which I've subscribed to for several years. The editor, Sharon Hudgins, had written an intriguing piece about how her two black cats, Branik and Flek, had developed a most unusual "craze for capsaicin." This intrigued me enough to call her at her home in Pittsburg, Camp County, Texas (located halfway between Dallas and the Arkansas border).

Our lengthy conversation was pleasant and cordial. She was extremely helpful in providing me what information she had on the matter, once I explained the purpose of my contact and this book project. I specifically asked why her two cats enjoyed playing so much with *fresh* habaneros, knowing how extremely hot they can be even to the stoutest human tastes let alone those of discriminating felines.

She remembered the incident well and admitted to being amazed the first time she and her husband discovered several of these fiery peppers lying on the kitchen floor with plenty of tooth and claw marks in them. This indicated to them that their furry friends had adequately sampled the volcano flavor of these habaneros besides playing around with them.

Ms. Hudgins laughed after giving one possible reason for this weird behavior: "Maybe my cats were just responding to their elevated testosterone levels, considering they're both adolescent males." But something else was at work here beyond mere sex-driven toms. Several times Flek had leaped on top of the kitchen counter to check out a variety of peppers that Sharon had left there. He didn't just content himself with sniffing them. No sirree! The critter went one step further and actually burrowed himself into the "colander full of fresh jalapeños, serranos, cayennes, manzanos, and habaneros." He soon emerged with the largest of all habaneros tightly clamped *between his teeth*!

"We couldn't figure out what was going on here," she continued. "We were at our wits' end and completely baffled by this mystery." So, she contacted Dr. Alice Wolf of Texas A & M University's College of Veterinary Medicine in College Station. Dr. Wolf is a professor in the Department of Small Animal Medicine and an authority on strange animal behavior. Upon hearing Ms. Hudgins's incredible tale, she, too, "laughed out loud." She told the magazine editor that "vets sometimes recommend smearing Tabasco sauce on an animal's bandages, to deter . . . chewing [them] off." These cats' love affair with the "chiles from hell" defied common logic.

However, both Dr. Wolf and Ms. Hudgins's own veterinarian, Matt Thompson, DVM, collectively suggested that it was probably due to a strong stimulation of endorphins that attracted these felines to the capsaicin. For the uninformed, "endorphins are peptides," the editor wrote, just a mix of different amino acids "which are secreted in the brain" and have a potent "pain-relieving effect" comparable "to that of morphine and other opiates."

Though there was no apparent external signs of physical pain, it may have been that Flek and Branik were feeling some kind of hidden emotional pain, such as loneliness or anxiety, which the capsaicin helped to alleviate through greater endorphin production.

Carrying Capsaicin One Step Further

Ms. Hudgins mentioned something else separate from her own cats' experience with chiles, but still indirectly connected. Ian Anderson is a flute player with the popular British jazz rock group called Jethro Tull. He lives in Scotland and grows habaneros year round in a specially built greenhouse located in his backyard. He picks and washes them before pureeing them in a blender and pouring them into containers to store in his freezer.

Several of his house cats have also been attracted to these chiles just as Ms. Hudgins's pair of black felines have been. And when one of them appeared not to be feeling well on a certain occasion, it managed to find enough strength to hop up onto the kitchen table where some of this habanero puree stood in a dish and to commence lapping a little of it. When the musician entered the room, this cat skirted away in haste. But by the next day, it seemed to have sufficiently recovered from its malady and was acting as perky as ever. (*Chile Pepper* magazine had scheduled an article on this man for later in the year, which necessitated that the editor interview him over the phone at his Scottish residence. This is how she came by way of this additional information.)

I was referred to Dr. Paul Bosland of the Chile Pepper Institute at New Mexico State University in Las Cruces. He is considered to be one of the best authorities on chile-pepper gardening. I was pleasantly surprised to discover that he didn't think the attraction of these felines for capsaicin to be unusual at all. In fact, he traded me a couple of true stories of his own. Several of them dealt with sick or injured dogs being seen by pickers in jalapeño fields eating some of these chile peppers right off the plants. A little while later the same canines were seen frolicking together and enjoying themselves as if they had been well all along. He also mentioned some dairy cattle that appeared unwell, eating roasted pepper skins and afterwards behaving in a normally healthy way again.

All of this anecdotal evidence seems to suggest that there is, indeed, medicinal virtue in the pungent constituent capsaicin. It has become a major ingredient in recent years in certain commercial liniments for the relief of human arthritis, muscle pain, and backache. It stands to reason, therefore, from the evidence previously given that capsaicin is also beneficial for pain relief in dogs and cats.

Ms. Hudgins wisely concludes her article by counseling readers: "DO NOT give peppers . . . to your own cats . . ." Instead, if capsaicin is to be administered to felines and canines it should be done in the form of a fluid extract or liniment. The liquid (ten drops) can either be squirted directly into the animal's mouth or mixed with some wet food. The liniment can be rubbed on those body parts experiencing the most pain.

Additional Herbs for Pain Relief

Several other botanicals I've found to be useful in pain relief are yarrow, mullein, and marshmallow root. These herbs constitute what I think are some of the best herbal measures for assuaging pain. There probably are others, but having worked with these, I can vouch for their success.

Teas are always better than capsules for promoting rapid healing. Liquids assimilate much more quickly than capsules do and their contents are more evenly distributed. The best way to make a tea is boil a pint of water and then add two teaspoons of any one of these three herbs. Stir, cover, and set aside to steep for 25 minutes. Strain and refrigerate. Reheat one-half cup and pour into a plastic container that has a one-and-a-half to two-inch spout on it. An empty mustard, catsup, or honey bottle or something similar is good for this. Open the animal's mouth and squirt the *warm* liquid directly into its mouth.

If capsules (usually five) are to be used, their contents should first be emptied and then mixed in with a little moist food. They are sometimes more convenient to use but usually not quite as effective as the teas are.

Pain Is a Complex Thing to Deal with

Managing acute or chronic pain in humans or animals is complex. This is because the pain and the perception of pain are realized at a number of different levels. These include the physical, the psychological, and the perceptual. Hence, there are many ideas floating around as to how pain might best be alleviated in man or beast.

Pain affects humans and animals in different ways. Such experiences can be related to factors such as age, gender, personality, and any previous experience with pain. Also, fear, stress, fatigue, and anxiety can depress the tolerance for pain. At the same time, rest, sleep, proper nourishment, good memories, healthy emotions, and diversion can boost pain tolerance amazingly well in people and pets alike.

The origins of pain are difficult to understand even for the most knowledgeable doctor or scientist. A simplified overview prepared for the reader may help provide him or her with a better idea of how it is transmitted. In the 1960s, Canadian and British scientists formulated the "Gate Theory" of pain. According to this hypothesis, pain signals excite a group of small neurons that constitute a pain "pool." When activity reaches a certain level, a presumed "gate" opens to transmit pain impulses upward to a human or animal brain. But large nerve fibers nearby can assist in regulating activity within the pool and keep the gate shut. Ice, heat, mechanical pressure, fruits, vegetables, herbs, nutritional supplements, and other things can stimulate those fibers and suppress the relay of pain messages.

A human or animal brain can, likewise, close this hypothetical "gate" another way by activating a descending pathway to block pain messages. Researchers speculate that brain-based pain control takes place when people or pets act heroically; they seem to disregard their personal pain, for example, the injured athlete who stays in a game or an arthritic dog bounding into a burning house through an open door to save his master's small child.

The herbs and nutritional supplements mentioned in this section are at least a beginning or point at which to start relieving the pain of a poor suffering creature. Animals are like us in this respect: They don't enjoy pain any more than we do, but have the remarkable habit of complaining a lot less than we do about it.

An Unusual Pain Treatment from Canada

Diana Petersen and her husband reside in St. Albert (close to Edmonton) in the province of Alberta, Canada. They have two purebred rottweilers named Wyllo (female) and Foli (male) that are two-and-a-half years of age. They also own two Persian-type cats, Jasper, a male, and Kandey, his female companion, both about three years old.

Sometimes Foli has a difficult time mounting or climbing down the stairs leading to the second floor of their large home. To relieve the pain of "his arthritic rheumatism" (as she prefers to call it), Diana employs a peculiar Chinese therapy known as moxa. A moxa stick looks something like a big cigar. It is lit and held in one hand, with the person frequently blowing on the end to keep it from going out. The idea is to apply this instrument next to the skin on certain acupuncture points and let the heat it generates penetrate into the body for no more than 45 seconds at a time.

"I hold the moxa stick in one hand," Diana told me over the phone, "while putting my other hand, fingers spread apart, next to Foli's body. I do this so I can feel the heat and know how close to hold the stick. I usually put it no closer than an inch to his fur. I use it on the hip joints, the knee joints, at the tail bone, and anywhere else my dog might be feeling pain. Following a few minutes' treatment of this, Foli is able to move around a lot better.

"I also give him a gentle thumb massage afterwards. I spread my thumbs and do circular motions down his spine and all the way to the end of his stubby tail. I repeat the process three or four times. It really helps to relieve his pain."

Acupuncture Relieves Pain too

With the permission of Dr. Bob and Susan Goldstein I've excerpted the following material from their November 1995 newsletter. My readers and I are indebted to them for this generous act.

"Acupuncture holds a special place in my heart because it has helped so many animals, and it opened the door for alternative medicine in many veterinary practices. It is the most widely available form of holistic treatment. Even if your veterinarian doesn't practice acupuncture, he or she is less likely to be critical of this alternative therapy.

"I remember the first time I saw acupuncture used on an animal. My brother, Marty, had recently received his certification. I was performing a routine surgery when the animal-health technician informed me that the dog was pale. Then, the dog stopped breathing. I was just about to instruct the technician to get the emergency drugs when Marty entered the surgery room with a small hypodermic needle in hand. He began working on an acupuncture point that I would later learn was called Governing Vessel 26 (GV26), which is located at the junction of the nose and lip.

"Marty inserted the needle and, instantaneously, the dog began breathing normally. His color changed from pale white to bright pink. The hospital staff and I stood there utterly amazed. After the surgery, the dog was up and about literally minutes later. Marty taught us all right then and there about GV26. Since that day, I have used this point about 10 times in emergency situations with excellent results.

"Allen Shoen, a friend of ours who is a veterinarian and an internationally renowned acupuncturist, describes similarly dramatic movements using GV26 and acupuncture in general in his book *Love, Miracles and Animal Healing* (New York: Simon & Schuster, 1995). Susan and I hooked up with Allen, joining him on several house and 'barn' calls."

"At a purely physical level, the insertion of a needle through the skin into a specific acupuncture point sets up a local inflammatory response. The immune system then springs into action releasing a number of beneficial chemicals including endorphins, the morphine-like compounds which relieve pain and inflammation. The treatment also stimulates the body's own cortisone. Acupuncture needles, by the way, are thin metal filaments. While the animal may feel a prick or flash of heat when the needle goes into a point, it doesn't hurt as you might think. While hypodermic needles used for medical injections are generally 21 or 22 gauge, acupuncture needles are much thinner, generally 28 to 31 gauge.

"The healing response, however, goes far deeper than the physical level. Hundreds of points have been painstakingly identified in people and animals. These points lie along vital energy pathways called meridians. The stimulation of the proper point or series of points balances the flow of energy through the meridians, producing healing effects elsewhere in the body. Likewise, improper stimulation of points can have mildly negative effects, which is why it's best to seek treatments from a trained, experienced professional.

"Acupuncture is a good therapy choice for just about any kind of pain with the exception of conditions where the pain serves as a diagnostic tool and where it's preventing the animal from doing additional damage. An example of the latter would be a slipped disc that is pinching the spinal cord. If the pain was removed, the animal may become overactive leading to complications. While the acupuncturist doesn't require a conventional diagnosis for treatment, you should always obtain a diagnosis from a veterinarian *before* using acupuncture.

"Acupuncture can be used successfully for painful conditions of the legs and spine, arthritis, Lyme's disease, inflammatory skin conditions, inflammatory conditions of the intestinal tract, constipation and diarrhea, even allergies, epilepsy and lung conditions, such as asthma.

"If your animal is currently under medical therapy for a painful or inflammatory condition, talk with your veterinarian about using acupuncture as an adju[n]ctive therapy or contact one of the veterinarians referred by the International Veterinary Acupuncture Society.

"Of the 56,000 veterinarians in the country, there are only about 500 certified veterinarian acupuncturists in the U.S. and another 500 worldwide. If your veterinarian does not do acupuncture or cannot provide a referral, you can receive a list of certified practitioners from the International Veterinary Acupuncture Society. Send a self-addressed, stamped envelope in care of Meredith Snader, VMD, 2140 Conestoga Rd., Chester Springs, Pennsylvania 19425. (The IVAS's Internet address is: IVASJAGG@ix.netcom.com)."

In a different issue a year later (marked only Special Supplement) they again reviewed acupuncture but with some additional data. "There is a technique that's similar to acupuncture, but that you can do at home without needles. Acupuncture involves needles inserted into specific points on the body. Acupressure uses pressure placed on these same points to stimulate the body. When the point is massaged, energy (the Chinese call this energy *chi*) is released and follows [the meridian pathways] to internal organs that are stimulated and revitalized thereby causing healing.

"There are other more subtle benefits. First by massaging your animal's body you are creating a physical bond with your dog or cat. Second, and probably more important, you are creating a positive mental and emotional bond with your animal which definitely aids healing.

"Let [us] give you an example and then a reference for you to follow for those who want to really get into acupressure. Suppose your dog or cat is suffering from stiffness related to arthritis of the front leg, specifically the elbow. The point you want to massage is Large Intestines 10 [LI-10]. This point is located on the outside of the front leg just in front of and below the elbow. Simply massage this point for 4–5 minutes every other day. If you're interested in learning more about acupressure, a great workbook is *Canine Acupressure* from Equine Acupressure, Inc. (303-841-7211). [By the way] the same points work for cats, too."

(The publisher of my many health books, Prentice Hall of Paramus, New Jersey, offers several good books on acupressure for human needs: *Body Reflexology* by Mildred Carter and Tammy Weber and *Acupuncture Without the Needles* by J. V. Cerney, DC, AB, DM, DPM. They can be ordered by mail or found in your local bookstore.)

Soothing Comfort from Aromassage

Aromassage is another natural healing process known to be of great help in the alleviation of pain discomforts. It isn't difficult to master, though not too many people may be aware of it. Anyone can do it on themselves or on their pets.

Aromassage is the mechanical hand movements side to aromatherapy which, I'm quite sure, more consumers have heard about than the other. It draws its strength from the essential oils contained in tiny glands on the outside or deep within the roots, wood, leaves, flowers, or fruit of an herb. This potent, aromatic substance is a concentration of the plant's own "life force."

In aromatherapy, the inhalation, external application, and baths are the chief ways in which such essential oils may enter a human or animal physical system. The oils themselves are highly volatile, evaporating readily on exposure to air. And when inhaled they may enter the body through the olfactory mechanisms of man or beast. When diluted and rubbed on the surface of the skin, essential-oil molecules permeate skin pores. Bath treatments, on the other hand, enable the pet or person to both inhale and absorb the oils via contact with the skin.

Once within the system, essential oils work to bring about harmony in those systems or organs that may be malfunctioning or are somehow out of balance. Think of aromatherapy and its accompanying aromassage as a "body tuneup" just as you might have a mechanical one done on your own car or truck. The aim here is for rebalancing and revitalization.

The essential oils common to aromatherapy are available at most health-food stores across the country. Making inquiries of those who are familiar with the various brands on the market will help you determine which ones are the best quality and most appropriate for your own or your pet's health requirements.

A type of massage called effleurage is probably the most useful movement in aromassage. It is a series of gentle, soothing strokes, which enable the essential oils to penetrate the body, producing almost immediate relaxation. I've adapted for this book some of the simple instructions given by Valerie Ann Worwood, an internationally recognized aromatherapist and reflexologist, who runs a clinic in her native Romford, England.

She suggests using "your whole hands" and "not just your fingers" in delivering "strokes that can be either long or short, firm or gentle." The result of such careful treatment is that the "muscles will be relaxed and nerve endings soothed, [the] circulation increased, [and] stress and tension relieved. Keep your hands relaxed but firm in this movement," she urges in *The Complete Book of Essential Oils & Aromatherapy* (San Rafael, CA: New World Library, 1991).

When working on the head of a cat or dog, always "put the oil on the fingertips and use the fingers, working all over the scalp." Never pour the oil directly on to the pet's cranium as this is apt to produce untoward reactions when it is immediately absorbed into the brain through the skin and muscle tissue.

To relieve animal headaches, "massage around the base of the neck and work upwards to the base" of the animal's head. Continue massaging here for about 30 seconds. Remember to use the fingers "in firm effleurage strokes to apply the appropriate essential oils."

When doing the neck of a household pet, be sure to "use small, firm circular movements, working from the base of the neck, either side of the vertebrae, to the base of the scalp. Work to the sides of the neck and repeat the movements, this time very gently, and work down again. Repeat several times with the appropriate essential oils."

Shoulder massage is done with both effleurage as well as petrissage strokes. (Petrissage is mostly done with the thumbs and always with *light,* never heavy, pressure. "Each movement should be slow and careful, never causing pain." Think of it as a gentle kneading of bread dough and you'll get the hang of it very quickly.) Work the shoulder muscles of cats and dogs using both types of massage movements along with the essential oils that seem most appropriate at the time. "Using your thumbs and palms, make firm strokes from the shoulder to the back" and return in similar fashion.

Doing aromassage on an animal's four legs helps it to walk and run better, as well as to break up fatty deposits located there. Massage upwards from the paws toward the shoulder blades of each leg, employing both effleurage and petrissage. But do this only on the fatty or muscular areas.

When doing the back of a household pet, either "firm or gentle effleurage or petrissage can be used. Do not massage over the vertebrae," however, Ms. Worwood cautions. "Start from the lumbar region of the back, and with two hands stroke all the way up to the shoulders. Slide the hands over the shoulders and return down the sides of the back" toward the animal's haunches. "Repeat this movement as many times" as deemed necessary. The longer the treatment, "the more relaxing it is" for your pet.

Doing the abdomen of a dog isn't so bad, but with a cat it can be a bit trickier. A cat doesn't automatically surrender its tummy side without having earned your trust and *wanting* to do so in the first place. Unearned trust or "not-in-the-mood" will quickly result in a "slash-and-bite" reaction if you're not careful. Use only circular movements, in a clockwise direction, in this region of the animal body. "Effluerage is the best stroke to use for this," Ms. Norwood recommends.

"*All* massage should be carried out with the flow of the body, that is, *toward* the heart," she adds.

I've worked out a plan schematic for which oils I think to be the most useful and appropriate for different parts of the animal body. They are listed in the following table according to body part:

Head	Lavender: Peppermint: Or use them on their own	3 drops 1 drop	Blend 1 drop of essential oil with 1 drop of olive oil
Neck	Ginger: Rosemary: Black pepper: Peppermint:	10 drops 10 drops 5 drops 5 drops	Dilute these essential oils with 2 tablespoons of extra-virgin olive oil
Shoulder	Ginger: Nutmeg: Chamomile:	10 drops 10 drops 10 drops	Dilute all three oils in 2 tablespoons of extra-virgin olive oil

Legs	Ginger:	10 drops	Dilute all four oils
	Clove:	5 drops	in 2 tablespoons of
	Nutmeg:	5 drops	extra-virgin olive oil
	Chamomile:	10 drops	
Back	Rosemary:	10 drops	Dilute all of these
	Marjoram:	10 drops	essential oils in 2
	Sage:	10 drops	tablespoons of
	Ginger:	10 drops	extra-virgin olive oil
	Basil:	10 drops	
	Eucalyptus:	10 drops	
Abdominal	Peppermint:	3 drops	Dilute all four
	Clove:	2 drops	essential oils with
	Thyme:	2 drops	1 teaspoon of
	Eucalyptus:	3 drops	extra-virgin olive oil

A simple and easy-to-follow book on the subject is *Aromatherapy: A Lifetime Guide to Healing with Essential Oils* (Paramus, NJ: Prentice Hall, 1997) by Valerie Cooksley.

PANCREATITIS

Saint Bernard's Wort: Natural Medicine for Cats and Cockatoos

On Saturday, October 18, 1997 Rob Goldberg attended a unique, first-of-its-kind Natural Care Animal Expo in the community of Old Westbury on Long Island, New York. In attendance were roughly 500 humans along with an assorted menagerie of dogs, cats, parrots, cockatoos, and several finches. He spoke briefly with Susan Marino, the conference organizer. "People are hungry for natural alternatives," she told him, as my friend sampled an organic dog biscuit.

"John, you would've loved it," he wrote in a lengthy letter received some weeks after the event. "I mean, there I was at this one booth and a guy was inserting two very thin acupuncture needles, one under each eye, of a golden retriever. I asked what this was for and he told me it was to 'improve the dog's nearsightedness.' His response made me want to knock on the top of his skull with my knuckles and yell into his ear, 'Hello up there! Anyone home?' I mean, how silly can you get?

"Of course, I know this stuff is right up your alley. But you gotta excuse some of my expressions. I like to think that I keep an open mind, but some things DO strain my credulity at times. Like the gal who was performing a 'laying on of hands' healing ceremony with a mangy gray cat so it could get in touch with, get this, ALL of its 9 lives! How about that for someone's elevator never quite reaching the top story? Maybe hers got stuck somewhere between ladies lingerie on the 5th floor and common sense on the 10th. What do you think?"

"The Cat Man Cometh"

Continuing with his interesting narrative, Rob, an artist by profession, mentioned something else that grabbed my attention. "There was this guy wearing a yellow-colored T-shirt that had an enlarged picture of a cat's head with the mouth opened imprinted on the front. Below it was boldly printed these words, 'The Cat Man Cometh.'

"Well, this got my curiosity, so I stopped to ask him the meaning of the message. He said his specialty was cats and *nothing* but cats! He claimed to be able to treat almost *any* kind of cat disease using nothing but plants. I jotted down his name and address and include it here in case you want to call him . . . it may be something or it may be nothing. . . . Just helping a pal out."

I called the number given me, which rang to a residence in the borough of Queens. "Bernie speaking," came the reply. I introduced myself and how I came by way of his name and number. He laughed and admitted, "Yeh, I'm the 'Cat Man.' What can I do for you?" I asked what herbs he used to treat feline pancreatitis. "Oh, that's an easy one," he chimed. "I thought maybe you was going to ask something more difficult."

He then proceeded to give me the herbal formula he used to treat cats suffering from pancreatic inflammation or swollen or fatty pancreas. "Take a quarter handful each—'bout one teaspoon apiece—

of dandelion root, yarrow herb, and nettle plant and add them to a small pan of boiling water—maybe not quite a quart (one-and-a-half pints?). Stir the herbs and slap a lid on that sucker. Turn down the heat and let 'em cook for, say, a few minutes. Then turn the heat off and let 'em awhile to cool. I strain only what I 'tend to use and leave the rest in the pan. I give, maybe 'bout a quarter cup to a sick cat a couple of times every day." He stated it should be room temperature and could be given "any ole way you want to." Here he wasn't that helpful, but I recommend using a turkey baster or empty syringe to fill with the liquid. Then grab the scruff of the cat's neck and gently bend its head back, which should cause the mouth to open.

"I usually do this for a week or until its condition 'pears to have improved some. But it always works, though we ain't talkin' 'bout an overnight mir'cle. Give nature time to do her thing an' she'll never fail ya."

The Cat Lady's Special Diet

We conclude this section with a simple diet prescribed by Anitra Frazier, the author of *The New Natural Cat* (see Appendix II).

PANCREATITIS DIET

3 cups chicken broth
2 cups cooked brown rice or barley or amaranth
1 cup raw peas
1 tablespoon bone meal or calcium lactate or calcium gluconate
2 organic eggs, separated
1 ½ cups raw liver chunks (preferably organic)
½ cup finely grated raw carrot or zucchini

Combine broth, cooked grain, peas, and egg whites in a pan. Simmer for 3 minutes. Turn off heat and add liver chunks. Cover and cool. Add bone meal, raw egg yolks, and remaining raw vegetables. Mix in a blender. Store one-cup portions (one day's supply) in resealable plastic bags or plastic storage containers in freezer. Thaw, as needed, by dropping bag (or standing container) in bowl of hot water. Serve ¼ cup servings 4 times a day.

PARALYSIS

Common Causes

Paralysis is more readily seen in dogs than in cats. It is more likely to occur as a result of disc problems in breeds such as dachshunds and German shepherds, but for different reasons. If the problem is due to a slipped disc, then massage and chiropractic manipulations will be of great assistance. If it is due to some form of arthritis, then treatment options will be limited to short fasting and a basic diet that will promote better health.

Occasionally, paralysis may be due to some type of injuries to the animal's spine or hips. If the head is banged in any way this could also eventually lead to temporary paralysis. It is not uncommon for blood clots to be implicated in this, too. If the cause isn't known and the paralysis appears to be severe enough, then by all means take the animal to a veterinary clinic at once for medical observation and treatment.

Whirlpool Therapy

It is a common practice in regular medicine to subject those who've suffered paralysis of some sort to whirlpool therapy in the belief that the constant rapid movement of the warm water will stimulate greater blood flow to inactive nerves and muscles. The same procedure may prove of some worth to a paralyzed dog or cat, but administered much differently, of course.

A veterinarian working out of the Midwest told me what he does in such instances. "I will put a large bath towel under the belly of the paralyzed animal. If it's of a larger size, then I will have an assistant help me. The pet is then carefully lowered into a tub or small pool of very warm water that is in continuous circulation. We will help it try to 'swim' around while holding on to the sides of the towel. We usually do about 15 minutes of this every day. Afterwards, one of us might give the animal a gentle rubdown on the spine and hips using a little peppermint oil. This keeps circulation coming into the area of the paralysis. We find that after a period of such treatments, the animal usually begins regaining some use of its limbs, however modest that movement may be at first."

He also utilizes fluid extracts of cayenne pepper and ginger root internally, which improves blood circulation. The herbal liquids are generally given directly through the mouth as quickly and efficiently as possible. "I recommend eight to ten drops for smaller animals and twice that amount for larger ones," he stated.

The Ritual of Bilberry

A woman named Martha O'Conner wrote me a lengthy letter one time on the many wonderful virtues of bilberry from her native Dublin. She told me a remarkable tale of curing her Irish setter's paralysis with this herb and vitamin E oil, but intertwined it with some local folklore history as well. Because her letter is so culturally enriching, I thought it would be appropriate here to quote in its entirety for the reader's general interest.

June 5, 1990
Dublin, Ireland

Dr. John Heinerman
Anthropological Research Center
Post Office Box 11471
Salt Lake City, Utah
United States of America, 84147

Dear Dr. Heinerman:

Please excuse the poor handwriting. But I hope you can make out most of what I'm trying to relate to you. I purchased a copy of your book *Heinerman's Encyclopedia of Fruits, Vegetables, and Herbs* (Englewood Cliffs, NJ: Prentice Hall, 1988) when I was in New York City recently. I'm enjoying it very much. But I noticed you didn't include bilberry.

This is a wonderful herb among the Irish. Let me share some of its history with you. Throughout the Emerald Isle there used to be celebrated for many centuries a festival called Lughnasa. It was usually held in the beginning of harvest every year in early August and named after the pagan god Lugh, in appreciation for providing rich crops.

Lughnasa was still being celebrated until just a few years ago in 195 different sites. About 95 of these were in mountain heights, ten were by lakes and five by river banks. Mountaintops have always been a favourite, though, often involving a journey that could take hours. Well, river banks and lakes were also chosen as sacred areas for these primal rites.

The festival varied from place to place and from generation to generation. The sacrifice of animals seems to have disappeared early in its evolution here, which I am truely grateful for as an animal lover myself. But many other elements still persisted through the centuries. There was always a solemn first cutting of corn or wheat, which the head of the family or the chief man of the community would offer to Lugh with a blessing. In my country here, where potatoes had taken the place of bread as the main food, a special meat from the first digging was eaten on La Lughnasa, the first day of the festival.

In return for these hilltop offerings, Lugh provided his people with the small dark blue bilberries that grew wild on the hillside. Picking bilberries is one of the longest lasting Lughnasa customs. The bilberries were looked on as a promise of the earth's fruitfulness and the bounty of the deity. It was so important for everyone to eat berries that they were taken home to those too old or weak to attend the festivities.

I hope I'm not boring you with too much of the history surrounding these Lughnasa festivities. Dancing seems to have been the most prominent and persistent element. Lughnasa dancing competitions were held in rural hamlets across Ireland. At Ganiamore in County Dongeal, where my parents live, for example, the prize for the best male dancer was his choice of bride from among all the female contestants. Dance songs were often sung acapella, so revelers needn't carry musical instruments on the long walk to the festival site. A boy or girl was selected to sing a song, which would pass from one to another until it was lilting enough to begin the dancing. Girls often wore bracelets and necklaces of bilberries, presents from their beaus. After the dancing, as twilight fell, the girls would leave their bilberry finery on the hillside as they made their way home.

The Lughnasa festival was so important in the lives of the Irish people and so involved with their ideas of welfare that Catholic priests and Protestant ministers could crush it. They had to either adopt it or permit it to continue in their versions of Christianity that they pushed upon our people.

Well, I've probably overdone as usual and given you too much of the folk history connected with bilberry. But figuring you are an anthropologist, I thought some of this you might find interesting.

What I really intended writing about was what bilberry and vitamin E oil did for my dog. Chester is a beautiful 8-year-old Irish setter. I noticed sometime ago that his usual gait was different. His hindquarters didn't seem to be functioning like they should, but I paid it little mind until one morning my dog couldn't even stand up. All he could do was raise himself part of the ways up with his front legs and then drag the back half of his body along very slowly. It was a pitiful sight to see and surely wrenched my heart.

Now I had heard from others how bilberry has been used in times past to assist older people who've suffered paralytic stroke. I reasoned that if it helped humans then why couldn't it help my dog. I obtained some *fresh* bilberries from a local market that sells fresh produce.

I measured out two-thirds of a cup and smashed them good with a large spoon. I added a tablespoon of liquid vitamin E and stirred everything together. Then I added this to some dry dog food, which I moistened with the liquid from some boiled mutton. Chester really likes the flavour of lamb and mutton and this encouraged him to eat more heartily. I gave this to him in the morning and again in the evening.

This was first done on a Monday. By Thursday, Chester was up and limping around. By Sunday he was slowly trotting again. And by the following Tuesday all traces of his paralysis had completely disappeared. I mentioned this treatment to a neighbor lady down the street from me, whose dog also suffered from some sort of paralysis problems. Within five days after bilberry treatment [the dog] was up and running around as usual.

There are other things that bilberry is good for. One veterinarian has used it to help some animals with eye disorders. And several physicians recommend it for improving vision in older people. You should include a section on bilberry when you write another herb book and mention the things I've written here.

May the "luck of the Irish" come your way.

Sincerely yours,

/s/ Martha O'Connor

(*Note:* The reader should consult Eye Disorders for more information about bilberry and the Product Appendix under Scandinavian Naturals for a popular and potent European bilberry extract known as Strix.)

PARASITES

Drinking Water on the Roof of St. Peter's Basilica

Jack and Marjorie Edwards are travel experts and write a weekly travel column for a major metropolitan newspaper in the city they live (which they asked not to be identified). Recently, they went to Italy and took a tour of the world's tiniest sovereign state, Vatican City, which is one-sixth of a square mile. This figures out to be about the same space as inside Minnesota's Mall of America in Minneapolis.

The Holy See, they informed me, houses one of the greatest complexes of museums anywhere. But these Vatican Museums must be approached rather like the running of a foot race. At least, your feet will feel that way after you've covered 26 miles or more on the complete circuit. Admission prices are roughly $9, which is a bargain for such an artistic and historical treasure trove.

During their lengthy tours, they took an elevator to the roof of St. Peter's Basilica. This is the world's largest Christian house of worship. To give you an idea of the height, let's put it in proportion with Egypt's oldest and most famous monument, the Great Pyramid of Cheops. That was built around 2600 B.C. and measures 479 feet tall from the base to its utmost pointed pinnacle. The Basilica, on the other hand, is only 452 feet high. In this instance, it seems the Pharaohs outdid the popes by some 27 feet and four millenniums (St. Peter's was completed in A.D. 1573).

The Edwardses told me that on top of the roof of the Basilica there were four public toilets. But not just any toilets, mind you. These rooftop facilities were Turkish toilets, those insidious holes in the floor flanked by porcelain footprints. Somehow, Jack said, "It seems almost a sacrilege to take a dump *on top* of the planet's greatest church." I noticed his wife give him a scolding glance of disapproval, perhaps thinking I was Catholic. Anyhow, he ceased speaking any more on that topic.

Marjorie then joined in and brought up the two drinking fountains. They were located adjacent to a bustling souvenir shop staffed by nuns. "Keep in mind, Dr. Heinerman," she reminded me, "that we're still talking about the rooftop of St. Peter's." Being thirsty, they opted for a drink of water. She brought out of a large travel bag they had with them two plastic coffee mugs and proceeded to fill them.

"The water stunk something terrible," she said with a frown.

"It was probably recycled urine," Jack gleefully volunteered. Marjorie gave him one of the those "wait-until-our-guest-leaves-dear-before-I-deal-with-you" kind of looks. Sensing that he was probably pushing matters a bit too far, he wisely and meekly retreated to humbler ground with an "I'm-s-sorry-sweetie" countenance and slightly bent head as a token of his presumed penitence.

Continuing forth in her dialogue, his wife declared: "I took from my purse some Agrisept and squeezed two drops in each of our cups before drinking. We had done this all through our trip and particularly in Rome where *everything* you eat, drink, or breathe is of questionable purity." As a result of doing this, neither of them contracted giardiasis and returned home without any unpleasant incidents of diarrhea.

I asked Marjorie what Agrisept was made of and she said, "It is a liquid extract of strong antibacterial components taken from the seeds of citrus fruits such as lemons, tangerines, and grapefruits."

Schnauzer Cured of Parasites

The couple had a little schnauzer dog excitedly running around their living room while I was visiting with them. Marjorie told me what had happened with "our dear little Sammie." "Our poochie started losing weight; her coat lost its luster and became dull; she developed diarrhea and became weak. Our vet told us Sammie had worms and wanted to give her some strong medicine to expel them, but I refused to go along with this.

"When I was having my hair done a couple of days later in the beauty parlor, my hairdresser told me about this product and where I could get some of it. So I took down the information he gave me and ordered a small bottle of it. I put two drops in every dish of Sammie's drinking water. Within eleven days she had lost most of her parasites and was beginning to feel and look better. After two weeks' treatment all evidence of intestinal parasites was gone according to our vet, who was totally baffled by the sudden turnaround but without any worming medications." (See Product Appendix under Calorad Support Group for more information.)

Another thing Marjorie has used this for is in the healing of external wounds. "Just spray some on the skin and see how quickly the problem goes away," she said.

(Also see under Diarrhea/Dysentery and Worms for more data.)

PAROVIRAL INFECTION

An East Texas Cure that Works

The canine parovirus type 2 (CPV-2) is quite common in breeding kennels, animal shelters, pet emporiums, and wherever pups are reared. Rottweilers, doberman pinschers, and English springer spaniels are reported to be at the most risk. Although the illness usually occurs in pups 6 to 16 weeks of age, it can strike at any age.

An herbalist friend of mine, Cheryl Jarman of Lufkin, Texas, related the following case to me by telephone recently:

"I had gotten a four-month-old puppy. It was an all-American cur cross, but mostly cur breed. Within 24 hours the dog became sick. It was running a high fever, passing blood in its stool, and vomiting excessively. I had tried all of the usual antibiotic shots prescribed by our local vet here, but nothing worked. I was desperate and didn't want to lose my puppy.

"I mixed together one teaspoon of powdered elecampane root and one-half teaspoon of the flowers, leaves, and stems of mixed mints, powdered ginger root, powdered echinacea, and powdered black-willow bark. I then poured two cups of boiling water over the mixture and let it sit in a covered pot for 30 minutes. I took a syringe (minus its needle) and drew 3 cc. of the strained liquid. I stuck this into the puppy's mouth and squirted the mixture down its throat.

"An hour later I increased the dosage a little more and kept this up every hour or so until night came. By the next morning our little female patient was drinking my herbal concoction right out of her bowl without any further force and eating for the first time in quite a few hours. The fever was gone and there was no further evidence of blood in her stool. She was kept off solids and given this mixture twice a day for four days. After this there was a gradual reintroduction to solid food again. Now she's just fine.

"Meanwhile, my next-door neighbor lost 10 of her 13 puppies to the very same infection. She faithfully followed the instructions of her vet and gave each of them the same standard prescribed antibiotics but to no avail. This is what happens when people put more trust in doctors and drugs than in the simple herbs that the Lord has created for the healing of man and animals."

Pet Therapy

Programs Going to the Dogs

In an insightful editorial in the medical journal, *Alternative Therapies* for July 1997, editor Larry Dossey, M.D., observes that there are "over 2,000 therapy programs throughout the United States" literally "going to the dogs." These canine therapists in their "gorgeous fur coats" with "enviable bedside manners, and cold noses" function strictly on a first-name basis. There is "Barlow, the 'hospice dog' at Riverside Methodist Hospital at Columbus, Ohio, and Pandora, who makes rounds in the critical-care unit at Maine Medical Center in Portland." Other four-legged therapists include "Max, Derby, Jake, and Kelly, who are part of the animal-assisted therapy program at the Rehabilitation Institute of Chicago."

Their owners bring them once a week to interact with different patients. Take the case of Marquette Buie, a young man who is recovering from gunshot wounds that left him a quadriplegic in 1994. "When I was hurting and thought I couldn't go on," he noted, "I'd come to see these dogs, and they did me worlds of good. They gave me a reason for wanting to continue living." Giving them verbal commands enabled him to regain the use of his voice, and tossing a rubber ball in a game of fetch helped him to learn to use his right arm, hand, and fingers, according to a short article in *The Journal of the American Medical Association* (274[24]:1897–1899) for 1995.

Pets Reduce Stress and Hypertension

The ability of pets to lower stress and help reduce blood pressure has been known for a long time among medical authorities. The work of Dr. Aaron Katcher and his associates at the University of Pennsylvania School of Veterinary Medicine is of particular interest here. They measured the blood pressures of dog owners while they were reading boring articles or books. They then took a second reading while these canine lovers were vigorously greeting their pets with pats, strokes, and words. The subjects' blood pressures were significantly lower during the greeting than during the reading.

Similarly, when individuals in a veterinary-clinic consulting room were talking to their pets, they had lower blood pressures than when they spoke with any member of the research team. Katcher and his colleagues also discovered that if people gaze into a tankful of tropical fish, it lowers their blood pressure, especially if it is already high to begin with. Katcher's work was featured in the journal *Continuing Education* (2[2]:117–21) for 1980 and the book *Interrelationships Between People and Pets* (Springfield, IL: Charles C. Thomas, 1981) edited by B. Fogle.

Pet Ownership and Heart Disease

A much heralded "pet-therapy" study conducted by Dr. Katcher and others appeared in the *Public Health Reports* (95[4]:308–12) for 1980. The research indicated a strong association between pet ownership and one-year survival in patients hospitalized with coronary heart disease, including heart attack. And this was even after accounting for individual differences in the extent of heart damage and other medical problems.

Katcher and the others also noticed that having a pet at home was a much better predictor of survival than was having a spouse or extensive family support.

Do Animals Really Care that Much About Us?

Animal concerns for human well-being are nothing short of amazing, as I have discovered in some 22 years of my own research. You needn't look any further for proof than an incident that grabbed world attention and garnered considerable newsprint space than what happened in mid-August of 1996. An eight-year-old Western lowland gorilla named Binti Jua, with a young one on her back, rescued a three-year-old boy who had fallen some 20 feet into the gorilla enclosure at the Brookfield Zoo in suburban Chicago, landing on his head. Heading off another gorilla, Binti picked up the child, cradled him in her arms, and placed him near a door where zookeepers could retrieve him. Water was sprayed on the other gorillas to keep them away. The boy was admitted in very critical condition to the Loyola University Medical Center, but was released within a week. Binti had been given stuffed, apelike dolls to play with in preparation for the birth of her baby, Koola. This was another instance where gorillas have sometimes shown maternal behavior to humans. Many of us remember the original Edgar Rice Burroughs's novel *Tarzan of the Apes,* which spawned a whole genre of books, comics, movies, and TV series over many decades. The principal theme there was about a young human infant being raised to manhood by a female gorilla.

An article in the London *Daily Telegraph* for April 4, 1996, showed how pets can sometimes double as doctors making house calls. A 45-year-old woman named Roz Brown of Cambridge fell into a potentially fatal diabetic coma. Holly, her West Highland Terrier, came to the rescue. Holly fetched a bag of "jelly babies" from behind a lamp on a coffee table, tipping two onto the floor with her nose, and then nuzzled Ms. Brown's head to rouse her. The sugary sweets revived Ms. Brown, who had suffered from diabetes for 38 years.

Another diabetes-related case was reported in the book *Everyday Miracle* (New York: Harper and Brothers, 1940) by Dr. Gustav Eckstein. A small spitz dog doubled every night as a night nurse for his mistress, who was a diabetic. Each night the canine would curl up in the angle of the woman's arm. He would immediately awaken and sound the alarm if her breathing pattern changed, "which is one of the telltale signs of ketoacidosis, one of the most dreaded complications of diabetes," Dr. Dossey noted in his previously cited editorial.

Pets Mend Broken Hearts

Not only do pets help turn around nearly impossible medical conditions for which doctors have almost given up hope, but they are able to mend broken hearts as well. Here are two true-life dramas that played themselves out in prison and in a hospital critical-care unit. And while both endings are sad, they nevertheless demonstrate the capacity of pets, *especially canines,* for bringing comfort to the final hour in the bleakest and most morbid conditions imaginable.

In March 1917 the roars of an impending revolution became imminent in Russia. This forced Czar Nicholas to abdicate the throne and move his family to exile in Tobolsk, Siberia. As the Bolsheviks kept a wary eye on him, his wife Alexandria (the granddaughter of England's Queen Victoria) and their four children, Anastasia, their youngest daughter, spent many hours playing with her pet spaniel. While the others frequently brooded on what might happen to them, this girl kept herself cheerful with the assistance of her wonderful animal companion.

In April 1918 the Bolsheviks ordered the Czar to report to Moscow, but instead hauled him and his family off the train and imprisoned them in a house in Ekaterinburg deep within the Ural mountains. Anastasia celebrated her seventeenth and last birthday in captivity, but even then she didn't despair. Her little dog had given her so much encouragement that she chanted prayers, sang hymns, sewed clothing, wrote letters, and daydreamed a lot.

On July 17, 1918, as the pro-Czar White Army attacked the Bolsheviks from the east, guards led the family into the basement. Anastasia accompanied them, clutching her dog in her arms. She watched in horror as her three sisters, younger brother, and parents were cut down in a rain of gunfire. Anastasia Romanov survived the initial shooting but was cruelly murdered with her dog in arms by the bayonet thrusts of the wicked executioners. The bodies were then burned, thrown into a mine shaft, and doused with sulfuric acid to prevent any possible identification.

Kathleen MacInnis, R.N., reported the following account in the *American Journal of Nursing* (91[7]:84) for 1991. She worked in the cardiovascular unit of Northern Michigan Hospitals in Petoskey, Michigan. At the time, she was caring for Dorothy, a young girl who was dying. Dorothy's blood pressure was sustained by intravenous medication, and her pain was managed with frequent morphine injections. What could the nursing staff do to make their patient's final hours more joyful?

They made the decision among themselves to have her beloved dog, Blackie, brought up to the floor for a short visit. Dorothy smiled in gratitude at their plans, but warned them in a very weak voice that her 18-month-old black Labrador was "wild and crazy" and could tangle everything up as he sniffed all over her room. When Blackie ventured into the coronary-care unit, his nails clicking on the tiles, he seemed fascinated by all the new smells. As he and a nurse slowly walked down the corridor, Blackie's healing magic came alive as people smiled at him and reached out to stroke his fur and pet him.

As they entered Dorothy's room, he took one crook-eared look at his mistress, gave one happy sniff, and climbed in bed beside her—burrowing in and snuffling his way from hip to armpit as he had learned to do previously. Dorothy was too sick to scratch his ears as she usually did. But she asked the nurses to do so, because she knew what Blackie wanted. "As we scratched his ears," Nurse MacInnis reported, "his eyes rolled partway back into his head in ecstasy; this pleased Dorothy the most." Later that week the young girl died in her sleep—following her visit with Blackie. "We felt very good about that," the nurse stated.

While both episodes have tear-jerking finales, their messages are similar. Both Anastasia and Dorothy were still in their maiden-hood when they died under very different circumstances. But at least they were comforted in their despair and cheered in their gloom by faithful dogs, which are truly "man's (and woman's) best friend."

Where to Solicit for Pet Therapies

There are currently only two nonprofit organizations that I know of that bring loving animals and people in need together for wonderful social interactions. These are Canine Companions for Independence (CCI) and Pet Partners, a division of the Delta society.

CCI was established in 1975 and has provided trained dogs for hundreds of people with various disabilities. They welcome volunteers or donations. Please contact them at 707-528-0830.

Pet Partners coordinates training programs that team animals and people to work in hospitals, nursing homes, schools, and reha-bilitation centers. Dogs, cats, birds, and even pot-bellied pigs are used in social interactive programs and more formalized therapy treatments. To find out more, or to make a contribution, please call Pet Partners at 1-800-869-6898.

PREGNANCY/BIRTH

Some Thoughts on Animal Pregnancies

Animal-care professionals such as veterinarians or shelter authorities are usually of the opinion that pets should be "de-sexed" so as not to be able to reproduce. The logic given for this kind of skewered reasoning is that there are way too many cats and dogs now without homes that must be destroyed every year. In her book *The New Natural Cat* (see Appendix II), author Anitra Frazier talked about the "situation horror" in New York City with its tens of thousands of footloose felines constantly falling prey to many wandering toms in search of a little *amour.* The result, she declared, is a "nightmare of unwanted kittens." She stated that in the Big Apple *every day* "hundreds of cats are destroyed," making little better than "trash [or] refuse!" Consequently, she is an outspoken advocate of neutering and spaying, saying, "it's the kindest way."

Organizations such as the American Kennel Club and many professional dog breeders lean in this direction, too, provided that purebred lines in different species are able to continue unchallenged without genetic contamination from cur mixes. "Mongrels should *always* be fixed," one top dog breeder told me. "And if not, then they should be *promptly* DESTROYED!" There certainly was no question in my mind where he stood on the subject.

But we must reckon with that great and first edict given by the Creator Himself in I Genesis 28 to the Preadamites and later on to Adam and Eve, when He commanded both groups to "Be fruitful, and multiply, and replenish the earth." And lest anyone misunderstood Him as to whom or what this applied, He included "every living animal that moveth upon the earth" at the very end of this same proclamation. There is no mystery connected with this at all. "Multiply and replenish" means just that, to give increase to one's own kind. Birth control, whether applied to humans or animals, completely circumvents this divine ruling and thwarts the very purposes of creation itself.

Well, there you have both sides of the spaying/neutering issue. These are merely thoughts to ponder and individually to act upon;

they are not necessarily absolutes. We make intelligent choices and live with the consequences; that is what life is all about.

Nutritional Fortification for Healthy and Easy Deliveries

The best guarantee to having healthy pups or kittens safely born to their mothers lies not so much in particular nutritional supplements given well in advance but rather in good and nourishing food. That's where the real promise comes in, determining how strong or weak the newborns will be and how trouble-free or difficulty laden each birth is.

There are obviously many variables connected with a normal and healthy birth. In his classic work *Dr. Pitcairn's Complete Guide to Natural Health for Dogs & Cats,* this veterinarian of many years' experience expounds at some length on the inherent problems connected with selective breeding. While this procedure has routinely produced pets that please us—"toy versions of dogs for lap companions; no-tail novelty cats"—it has also "led to [many] defects and malfunctions" along the way. "So many of the features we find appealing in purebred animals are actually the products of arrested development—either physical or psychological," Dr. Pitcairn acknowledges. And "inbreeding . . . to fix a given characteristic in a breed" only exacerbates the problem. For instance, he notes, "miniature poodles bred for just the right color have produced litters in which the puppies had severely malformed lower jaws." When this kind of genetic tinkering happens there will always be repeated birth defects, no matter now natural or organic the female animal's diet may have been.

Then there is the matter of the commercial dog foods. Responsible veterinarians (and their involved spouses), such as Dr. Robert and Susan Goldstein and Dr. Richard and Susan Pitcairn, have made almost lifetime careers of denigrating commercial dog foods in nonlitigious language. Their unified goal has been to warn pet owners everywhere of the inherent health dangers present in lifetime feedings of these products to the four-legged companions they cherish. Unnatural, unwholesome, and nonnutritious food does not make sound puppies or well kitties. In fact, just the opposite is true: Nutritionally deprived staples invariably result in young animals that thrive poorly. The yardstick by which to measure a healthy litter is "quality food for the mother yields quality offspring," plain and simple.

Throughout this book are scattered numerous recipes, all of which ultimately promote health and well-being in cats and dogs. The reader is encouraged to take the time to read the entire text and become acquainted with all of them. Some are located in specific sections relating to nutrition, such as Diet Tips. But others are less observable, such as the health-giving recipe under Distemper. But speaking collectively rather than individually, I've singled out some food sources that should be included in the diets of every pregnant feline and canine in order for them to have bright, beautiful, and energetic newborns.

- Whole grains (these should be lightly cooked)
- Raw vegetables (grated or juiced)
- Cooked vegetables (lightly steamed or baked)
- Enzyme-rich substances (low-fat yogurt)
- Mineral-rich items (tuber vegetables)
- Vitamin-rich foods (some fresh fruits and fruit juices)
- Adequate protein (selected meat cuts, eggs, and cheese)
- Omega 3 and 6 fatty acids (fish and fish oils, flaxseed and sun-flower-seed oils)
- Dietary fiber (grains and vegetables)
- Trace element sources (certain seaweeds and organ meats)
- Pure water (spring, filtered, or distilled)

While addressing the subject of nutritional fortification, I'd like to include a few others usually not associated with nutrition per se: love, kindness, patience, gentleness, and devotion. All of these virtues may be considered "nutrients from the soul," which nourish the animal heart and mind and contribute to its overall emotional health and mental well-being.

There you have it in a nutshell—things to feed and things to show an expectant mother cat or dog for healthy babies and normal deliveries.

Helpful Meals for Healthy Gestations

I'm grateful to Dr. Bob and Susan Goldstein for allowing me the use of three of their favorite recipes borrowed from a Special Health-Booster Supplement issue of their monthly newsletter *Love of Animals.*

PROTEIN DINNER

1 cup brown rice

1 pound organic liver (use organic chicken or lamb if organic liver isn't available

1 grated carrot (organic)

1 cup watercress, finely chopped

1 tablespoon dandelion greens, chopped

1 small beet, grated

1 clove garlic

½ teaspoon ground kelp

4 springs parsley, finely chopped

1 teaspoon flaxseed oil

1 egg yolk, organic

Cook the brown rice in two cups distilled or filtered water until soft and all the water is absorbed. Steam the liver until browned on both sides. Cut up fine and mix well with vegetables and rice. Add egg yolk and mix again.

AS MEAL

Cats and small dogs (1–12 lbs.)—½ cup twice daily
Medium dogs (15–35 lbs.)—1 cup twice daily
Large dogs (50–85 lbs.)—1 ½ cups twice daily
Giant dogs (85+ lbs.)—2 cups twice daily

VITAMIN-MINERAL-TRACE ELEMENT LUNCH

8–10 medium organic potatoes, unpeeled
2 cloves garlic
1 inch ginger root, chopped
4 organic carrots with tops, cut into 2-inch pieces
2–4 leaves kale, or dandelion greens
8 large sprigs parsley
1 large beet, quartered
½ organic chicken
½ teaspoon kelp

Put all ingredients in stewpot. Cover with distilled or filtered water. Bring to a boil, then cover and let simmer for an hour. You can feed the full stew (debone the chicken), or just add the [nutrient]-rich strained broth with the chicken to your natural base food.

AS MEAL

Cats and small dogs (1–12 lbs.)—½ cup twice daily
Medium dogs (15–35 lbs.)—1 cup twice daily
Large dogs (50–85 lbs.)—1 ½ cups twice daily
Giant dogs (85+ lbs.)—2 cups twice daily

FIBER-FATTY ACID-ENZYME SNACK

This light meal is nutritious and easy on your animal's digestion. This meal is a treat for [our pets].

2 cups flaked organic groat or oatmeal
1 large organic apple, finely chopped
½ teaspoon raw red-clover honey (optional)
1–2 tablespoons ground-up almonds
2 tablespoons organic plain low-fat yogurt

Cook the oats according to the package directions, then let them cool. Add the rest of the ingredients and mix well. Feed 3–4 times a week as a treat, or mix it with a natural-base food as a topper.

AS MEAL

Cats and small dogs (1–12 lbs.)—½ cup twice daily
Medium dogs (15–35 lbs.)—1 cup twice daily
Large dogs (50–85 lbs.)—1 ½ cups twice daily
Giant dogs (85+ lbs.)—2 cups twice daily

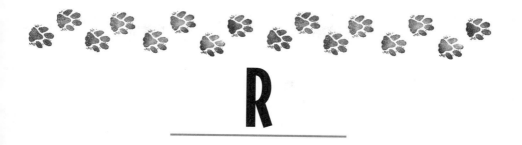

R

RABIES

A Morning to Remember

In North America, four strains of viral polioencephalitis are endemic in their respective populations: fox, raccoon, skunk, and bat. All four strains can be transmitted to dogs and cats very easily. I'd like to share a close call I had with the latter some years ago.

During the time that Jake the office cat had the run of the Anthropological Research Center (of which I've been the director for 23 years), there were several occasions that bats managed to get into the building where we were then located. It was an older structure, built in the late 1890s, and was—how should I say?—rather airy and drafty in places it probably shouldn't have been.

One night after working my usual nine-to-nine shift, I turned off equipment and lights, bade my little furry friend "good night," locked up, and went home. In the morning, I got a call from several panicky secretaries who insisted that I come down *"immediately"* in very definite tones of voice. Not knowing what the problem might be, but assuming it was probably of an urgent nature, I hastily drove to the office.

Both women pointed to a dead bat on the carpeted floor in the middle of one room. Directly in front sat Jake on his haunches, flicking his tail and occasionally meowing. The secretaries were absolutely petrified of both, believing that the dead bat was rabid and that somehow my cat had contracted it and was now acting crazy himself.

I put on some work gloves, picked up the bat by its wing, and put it into a large mailing envelope, which I sent out to a friend who worked at a toxicology laboratory, to check for rabies. A telephone call received later that afternoon indicated we had nothing to worry about. Jake was just being his usual but strange self and, thankfully, wasn't infected with anything serious. But that was a morning to remember, for sure.

Danger Signals

When polioencephalitis virus enters the bloodstream due to a bite from a rabid animal, it quickly travels to the brain where severe tissue inflammation sets in. This results in some bizarre personality and behavioral changes.

- An infected animal may seek solitude, whereas before it may have enjoyed being around people.
- Dissatisfaction becomes evident. A formerly confident and friendly animal may now turn apprehensive, nervous, and anxious.
- Extreme mood swings are prevalent. These can range from sudden shyness to frightening aggression.
- Other erratic behavior is readily apparent. An infected animal may suddenly snap or bite, lick or chew a wound, bite its leash or cage bars, and tend to wander about aimlessly.
- An infected creature will demonstrate excitability, irritability, and uncharacteristic viciousness.
- As the disease progresses, muscular incoordination, disorientation, seizures, and paralysis quickly set in.
- There is a change in tone of bark or meow.
- Excess salivation or frothing is noticed.

Infected animals manifesting any of these symptoms present a clear danger not only to themselves and other animals, but also to their human owners and family members. *Under no circumstance* should an individual attempt to deal with such an animal *alone*. It is always best to have someone else present, especially someone who knows what he or she is doing if the owner doesn't. Gloves, boots, a heavy coat, and leash are almost necessary equipment when attempting to handle a larger animal. Preferably, a veterinarian should be involved, if one can be found who won't rush to judgment and suggest that the animal be promptly put to sleep.

Treatment Not Impossible

In his book, *Dr. Pitcairn's Complete Guide to Natural Health for Dogs & Cats* (Emmaus, PA: Rodale Press, Inc., 1995; p. 325), the author states with some reservations that such infected animals "can be treated with homeopathic medicine, but sometimes with difficulty." Following a natural course of treatment with a legally required rabies vaccine almost always spells doom for a recovered animal, he observes.

In my tenth book (I've written some 55 of them as of 1977) entitled *Healing Animals with Herbs* (Provo, UT: BiWorld Publishers, 1980; pp. 61–64), I devote several pages to a remarkable plant that has served as a perfect antidote to rabies for a couple of centuries. It is elecampane root and will alleviate the symptoms of rabies in man and beast alike if administered early enough in the form of a liquid.

I present ample evidence from a number of different sources to show how effective a remedy it is for something as serious as polioencephalitis. One case, in particular, stands out as a fine example of what this simple herb can do. "Two men living near [Philadelphia] were bitten in the hand by the same dog, and within fifteen minutes of each other. The dog, a stranger to them, was secured and imprisoned to await an owner. The next day he showed unmistakable signs of madness. . . ." The owner came and was permitted to administer some elecampane decoction to the afflicted dog. It was closely watched and all signs of its hydrophobia disappeared.

"Alarmed for their [own] safety, both men came to the city [of Philadelphia] and [sought out the services of an eminent] physician. . . . He prescribed [for them] elecampane root. One of the men remarked, 'That is an old woman's remedy,' and refused to take it. This man returned to his home, placed himself under the care of his own doctor, who cauterized the wound, and administered medicine to salivate him. On the ninth day he was seized with spasms and died in [great] agony.

The other and more fortunate man took the elecampane as prescribed and never suffered in the least degree from the dreaded disease."

Elecampane root is abundant in the fields and waste places of eastern North America, growing from Quebec to the Carolinas and Georgia. The fibrous, top-shaped rootstock is brown on the outside with a creamy white interior. It is available through some health-food stores or can be ordered by mail from Indiana Botanic Gardens (P.O. Box 5, Hammond, Indiana 46325; 219-947-4040).

The liquid form is the best way to take this root. Put two table-spoons of coarsely cut, dried elecampane root in a stainless steel pan. Add one pint of milk and bring almost to the boiling point. Reduce the heat to a lower setting and simmer, covered with a lid, until only one cup of milk remains. Strain this liquid through a sieve and refrig-erate. Take two to three tablespoons every couple of hours, eating no solids but being sure to drink plenty of water. For an infected ani-mal I advise confining it to a cage and pouring the entire contents into its water dish where it may have easy access to the tea.

Wheat-grass or barley-grass powder is also helpful. In between the doses of elecampane, the sick animal can be served some of this chlorophyll. Stir one to two tablespoons of either cereal grass in two cups of cool water and pour into the animal's food bowl. Chlorophyll is especially good for providing energy to physical sys-tems weakened by disease and for stimulating the immune defens-es into action. (See the Product Appendix under Pines International.)

And, by all means, don't forget vitamins C and B-complex. Vitamin C is critical for fighting infections and the B vitamins assist in regulating nerve transmissions. Also, yarrow herb is excellent for tissue inflammation. It can be administered in the form of a tea with good results.

RED EYE

The Causes

About every case of red eye fits into one or several of the following categories: inflammation of the eyelids (blepharitis); conjunctivitis (see entry for it elsewhere in the text); inflammation of the cornea (keratitis); inflammation of tissues overlying the sclera (episcleritis) and inflammation of the sclera (scleritis); inflammation of the iris (anterior uveitis); glaucoma; hemorrhage in the anterior chamber of the eye (hyphema); infection of the eyesock (orbital disease).

Scottish Treatments

Back in the first quarter of 1979, I received from a friend in Scotland a newspaper clipping telling of the highlights of a public lecture given by one Theron Dunkirk, designated only as "a small animal practitioner" by the *Glasgow Herald,* which reported the curious event.

While the majority of this article has already been reproduced under another entry (see Conjunctivitis) earlier in the text, a few more paragraphs are inserted here for the reader's benefit. The story focused mostly on different remedies that the gentleman claimed were good for various ailments of the eyes in animals. The paper mentioned as follows:

> Mr. Dunkirk wisely observed that small animals were "less likely" to experience ocular traumas of this sort if their residential environments were kept clean and orderly. He was of the decided opinion that hyperemia could be just as easily treated with medicinal plants as with drugs such as atropine or aspirin.
>
> His very favorite herbes for this were rose petals, lilies, summer savory herbe, and rue flowers. He preferred to steep everything in spring water over several days time without the benefit of heat. He believed that by cooking them, their wonderful medicinal virtues disintegrated rapidly.
>
> The herbes and flowers could be lightly crushed with a mortar in a stone pestle and then transferred to a flask before the cool water was poured over them. After it was corked, the contents should be allowed to set a few days undisturbed before being strained off.
>
> The red eyes of small animals could then be frequently bathed with this solution until the condition had cleared up. Of this Mr. Dunkirk was most certain.

Other remedies include using nonalcoholic liquid extracts of either chickweed herb, couchgrass rhizome, or eyebright herb. (See Product Appendix under Nature's Answer for more information.) Also a boric-acid solution obtained from any pharmacy works just as well.

Ringworm

Ways of Fighting the Ringworm War

Shirley Moskowicz of Truth or Consequences, New Mexico, had barely introduced her *sixth*—you read it right the first time—Siamese cat to her household when she and the rest of her cats all came down with ringworm. "I was beside myself as to what to do," she bemoaned this unhappy event to me by phone recently. "I frantically called a dermatologist and the first thing he asked me was 'Was your new cat a kitten?'

"As I was soon to learn, this is a very common problem. The doctor gave me some pills, which he said was the most effective way to treat someone suffering from multiple lesions, as I was. I think it was Griseofulvin. It helped a little, but also gave me headaches and diarrhea, and made my abdomen become bloated.

"I decided to treat my own body after this, figuring I couldn't do any worse than the doctor had done with me. I made a liquid mixture consisting of one-quarter teaspoon each of the liquid Japanese aged-garlic extract, goldenseal-root tincture, and lime juice. I massaged some of this on those parts of my scalp and skin that were afflicted with fungus. I did this several times a day. Within four days there were no more signs of itching or irritation."

She took all of her cats to a local veterinarian who specialized in alternative treatments and rejected most synthetic drugs. The first thing he did was to clip away all of the area around the infected, bald spots. He was careful in his disposal of the hair, making sure to burn it in an incinerator located outside his clinic. He also vacuumed up the area where the clipping had been done and had an assistant scrub down the table on which each of the cats had lain. During the entire course of treatments he always wore plastic gloves. He told her that such precautions were absolutely imperative because of ringworm being such a contagious disease.

He then made a special preparation of lemon juice, powdered cabbage leaves, and expressed garlic oil, which was liberally applied to every infected patch of skin of each cat with a basting brush. He instructed her to continue doing this every other day until no new lesions were evident. Within a matter of weeks the problem was finally corrected. "*No* drugs were used at all," she said with an obvious tone of pride in her voice.

The veterinarian explained to her how to make more of this preparation at home when needed. She squeezed the juice from two fresh lemons into a small container. She bought and used a garlic press to extract the oil from six small peeled garlic cloves. This was added to the lemon juice and stirred thoroughly. Next, she cut a head of green cabbage in half, removed the core, and then stripped off the leaves and laid them flat on several cookie sheets. She put them in an oven set somewhere between 220° F. to 250° F. and left them there for several hours until they had thoroughly dried. After this, she reduced the leaves to a fine powder in a mortar and pestle. Approximately one level teaspoon of this cabbage powder was then added to the liquid mixture.

"It was a little tricky in the beginning," she said, "working with this stuff. If too much powder was used, it would make the mixture a thick glop that wouldn't spread evenly. I finally got it right so that the consistency was fairly even and still rather liquid."

Later on, a friend of hers who also kept some cats (but not as many), mentioned what she had done for the ringworm problem in her pets. She clipped the hair away from the infected parts and dabbed on some tea-tree oil from Australia. But, she added, melaleuca and eucalyptus oils could also be substituted if the other wasn't readily available.

I've also heard of others adding one-half teaspoon zinc gluconate powder, one teaspoon of lecithin granules, and one teaspoon of cod liver oil to their pets' food for this problem. While these things don't kill the fungus, they certainly help the skin to recover more quickly.

(See also Itching.)

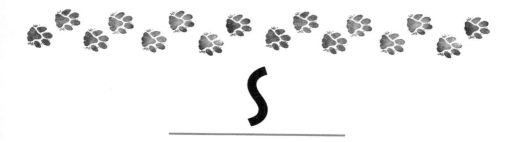

SKIN PROBLEMS

Recognizing Skin Irritations

Skin disorders are quite common in cats and dogs alike. They are relatively easy to detect. A pet owner should look for unusually dry skin; white, scaly patches resembling dandruff; large brown flakes; evidence of redness, itching, crusty scabs, blisters and pimples between the toes; skin discoloration; skin odor; greasy hair and some hair loss; chronic inflammation inside ear canals (as well as beneath the ear flaps on dogs); swollen glands; occasional diarrhea; and foul-smelling, sometimes bloody urine.

Veterinarians have differing opinions on what may cause such disorders. Richard H. Pitcairn, DVM, the noted author of *Dr. Pitcairn's Complete Guide to Natural Health for Dogs & Cats* (Emmaus, PA: Rodale Press, Inc., 1995; p. 304) lists toxicity, suppressed disease, and mental/emotional disturbances as likely reasons for this. On the other hand, Charles E. Loops, DVM, blames poor diet and particularly vaccinations in an enlightening article on the subject which appeared in the May/June 1997 issue of *Natural Pet Magazine*. He claims that "a vaccine . . . consist[ing] of five to seven viruses injected directly into the bloodstream [can] wreak havoc with [an animal's] immune system." The effects won't show up immediately, but will appear down the road in successive generations.

Treatment Tips

Skin problems are generally complex and require multifaceted approaches. There are some simple things that a loving pet owner can do. But it should be emphasized here that the skilled services of a knowledgeable veterinarian may also be needed in order to effect a complete cure of the problem. Using both systems of treatment will guarantee a more speedy and proper recovery than if either one were used by itself.

While it is my intention to provide greater detail to some of the more natural methods, I want to say a few words in regard to homeopathic preparations, which have become extremely popular of late in treating human and animal conditions. Granted that they are effective to some extent. But I've never felt too comfortable with them in general. I honestly believe that homeopathic agents are way too close to conventional drugs and, therefore, potentially harmful to human or animal bodies down the road. I respectfully submit that homeopathy isn't as natural as it seems. Nor is it a system of healing divinely approved or inspired.

Give up vaccinations for good, both for your family and the pets you have around. Do this in spite of advice to the contrary from your pediatrician or veterinarian. Both my brother and I were raised without the benefits of such immunizations. And the various dogs and one cat I've had in my life were never vaccinated either. I truly think that all of us were better off without them and certainly a lot healthier.

Change the diet of your pet. Switch to fresh food at least four times a week, using raw meat and organic vegetables. And feed your cat or dog only the best commercial foods that contain no by-products or chemical preservatives. Train yourself to be more of a label reader and spend more time scanning the finely printed list of ingredients before purchasing your next pet foods. Add supplements to provide the necessary vitamins and minerals that are lacking in our nutritionally depleted soils.

One of the best measures of relief to pets suffering from skin problems is to bathe them with a nonirritating soap once or twice a week (obviously less for cats, who despise getting wet). Consider brewing up a batch of green tea and letting it cool. Then strain it and sponge those afflicted parts of your pet with it. You'll be amazed at how healing the tannic acid in this tea solution will prove to be.

Between baths, you can smear these areas two or three times a day with the gel from a fresh aloe-vera leaf. Cover them with tape if your pet begins to lick it off. Commercial preparations of aloe-vera gel are available from health-food stores. Ironically, aloe vera is one of the simplest and most effective remedies for a wide variety of skin ailments, but is often overlooked in preference to fancier products because it's so ordinary and lacks the marketing pizzazz that the others seem to have.

Finally, a little animal psychology is in order here. As strange as it may seem to some, a pet's skin problems could be inadvertently linked to boredom, frustration, anger, hostility, and loneliness. Study your pet more carefully, watch the eyes and body language, and look for signs of these emotions. Then take the appropriate steps to correct such factors.

A Mild Food Fast

Many years ago, as a young boy growing up in Provo, Utah (home to Brigham Young University), I became acquainted with an old veterinarian named Dr. Arthur Vance. He was an octogenarian and knew a great deal about animals and how to treat them. He helped correct a skin condition from which my first animal—a German shepherd named Flame—was then suffering. The dog had what veterinarians sometimes refer to as "hot spots." These are patches of an animal's skin that become severely inflamed, though in good condition otherwise.

I remember Dr. Vance telling me after looking my pet over, "If he was living out in the wild, he would follow his basic wolf instincts and avoid food for six or seven days. All creatures in the wild have enough sense to do this when they don't feel good. It's only when they get domesticated and have food put before them all the time by doting masters that they lose this sense of fasting."

He went on to explain how a simple fast would enable Flame's system to do some internal housecleaning and throw off any debris that may have accumulated from constant eating. Fasting would also give his digestive tract a much needed rest, while the rest of his body began the slow process of healing itself again.

I was to slowly introduce my dog to this fast for a couple of days by feeding him some cooked oatmeal over which had been poured a little beef broth instead of milk. (Milk could be used for cats, however.) I was to alternate this with two small boiled potatoes (quartered and unpeeled) that had been lightly seasoned with a pinch of sea salt and moistened with a tiny amount of beef broth. (The beef broth could be obtained by simply boiling some beef bones obtained from the meat section of any supermarket. And, in the case of cats, fish bones can be boiled to make a delicious stock for them.)

Days three and four were to consist of boiled cabbage, carrots, turnips, and beets. He recommended that I only *partially* cook these vegetables and to do so in beef broth rather than in water. In his own 60 years of veterinary practice he found that this appealed more to animals' finicky tastes than did cooking such items in plain water. Nothing was salted since the beef broth itself had sufficient salts in it for flavor. (One would merely substitute some clear fish broth for beef broth when administering the same program to cats with skin problems.) There was to be *no more meat* after this for the duration of the fast.

The fifth, sixth, and seventh days were to be nothing but *liquids*. Dr. Vance detested tap water, declaring that the chlorination and fluoridation poisoned rather than helped animals in the recovery stages. I was to use only well or distilled water. *Freshly made* tomato juice was his favorite base to work from. We had an old Osterizer in the kitchen, which I used for this purpose. I usually started with a couple of medium-sized and *ripe* tomatoes, adding a tiny bit of water to thin things down if the mixture became too thick. Then I would add a little parsley *or* spinach leaves *or* turnip leaves *or* Romaine lettuce. For an animal, he didn't believe it was necessary to have more than just one chlorophyll source at a time. If my dog didn't immediately take to this juice, I was advised to substitute a little beef broth in place of the water.

A one-week mild food fast was adequate for a dog the size of my German shepherd, he told me. In the beginning of the second week I was to gradually bring my dog out of it by working backwards with the same program. That is to say, I started giving Flame small portions of different vegetables again, cooked in beef broth. The last few days consisted of simple cereal grains, some scraps of lean meat, and some beef bones. *Under no circumstances* was I to give him any canned or dried dog food during this nearly two-week recovery program.

I must admit that as a boy of 12, I was a bit skeptical that this strange regimen would work. But I followed the old gent's directions and was happily surprised to see my dog's skin irritation virtually cleared up by then. This man had won over a young boy's trust, and he became one of my heroes in early life.

Other Remedies that Work for Cats

A girl I knew by the name of Beverly had a female cat that was her pride and joy. She fussed over her a lot, frequently brushing the fur and tying variously colored ribbons about the animal's neck in small, fancy bows. As boys, some of us used to make fun of her for devoting so much time and attention to the cat. But she ignored us, as girls and women are good at doing with the opposite sex, and went about her business as if we didn't exist.

But there came a time when her cat got one of these "hot spots." It differed from the one my dog had in that the irritated skin discharged a yellowish pus that smelled awful. Beverly was beside herself and didn't know what to do. I told her about Arthur Vance, and she asked me to take her and the cat there. We walked a number of blocks to where he lived. The retired vet examined her feline for a few minutes, and then made the following recommendations, as near as I can recall.

Beverly was to clip away the hair surrounding the infected area. Then she was to bathe *only* this portion of skin with a very mild hand soap. The area was to be thoroughly rinsed with some cold black tea and left to dry in the air. Several times a day she was to wash the immediate area with cotton balls soaked in a weak solution of boric acid. Afterwards, some Rex's Wheat Germ Oil was to be applied on the surface several times a day. (This is where I first became acquainted with this animal-strength vitamin E oil, which our family has faithfully used for many human and animal needs for nearly four decades. A quart costs $65 and may be ordered from Anthropological Research Center, P.O. Box 11471, Salt Lake City, UT 84147.)

Beverly was also instructed on how to conduct a mild food fast with her feline. I assisted her a little with this until she got the hang of it. In nine days the problem disappeared and all nine lives of her cat enjoyed good skin health again.

As I grew older and became more interested in natural healing, thanks to my grandmother Barbara Heinerman and people like Arthur Vance, I discovered the properties of other herbs that worked well for different skin problems, both in humans and in small animals.

Stinging nettle, in powder and liquid forms, has always been a favorite of mine. It works especially well for acne in youth and for tiny pimples that show up in the faces of pets. A strong solution of the tea is practical for bathing the face several times a day. Also, small dabs of the powder applied directly with a cotton swab to cysts or pimples and left there for a few hours will help to dry them out.

Cabbage and garlic are useful, too, but in a different way. They should be given internally in small amounts and best mixed with a little lean meat or beef broth to improve their flavors for finicky eaters. Their high sulfur contents tend to expedite skin healing from within by attacking any bacteria, viruses, or parasites that may be partly responsible for the skin problems in the first place.

I've always been a big fan of the trace element silicon. It occurs abundantly in horsetail as well as in homeopathic tissue-cell salts. Empty one capsule of the powdered herb into a cat's food or two capsules of the same into the chow of a large dog twice every day for up to a week until the skin problem shows change and improvement.

Goldenseal root is another big favorite with a number of holistic veterinarians. Some of the powder can be mixed with a little water and applied by cotton swab directly onto irritated skin that is discharging purulent matter. Wild Oregon grape is also good for this. Both herbs share the single constituent known as berberine, which not only is strongly disinfectant and antibiotic, but also serves as a coloring principle to give both their golden-yellow hues.

Kelp is probably an odd thing to include here, seeing as how not too many veterinarians or pet owners are sold on it. But this happens to be one of the richest sources of iodine that I know of. And iodine is particularly important for stimulating underactive thyroids in many animals. Hair loss and skin problems are sometimes linked to glandular imbalances in the endocrine system, and kelp is just the ticket for normalizing things again. I suggest using the granules and sprinkling some over the food of your pet every day for as long as necessary.

A small, potted aloe-vera plant is always good to have on hand for minor skin irritations. A piece of this succulent herb can be cut off and its gel squeezed onto the afflicted area for prompt relief of itching and reduction of inflammation. Aloe vera is such a common plant that I'm surprised more pet owners don't keep one or several around the house for treating cutaneous problems. While some aloe-vera products may serve the purpose to some extent, there is really no substitute for the genuine article. Investigate this plant further and you'll find it's an ideal agent for treating many types of skin afflictions.

SPAYING/NEUTERING

Bob Barker's Traditional Sign-Off

For almost 30 years Bob Barker has been the beloved host of America's most popular game show, *The Price Is Right*. At the end of every segment, he has signed off with the traditional line: "This is Bob Barker reminding you to help control the pet population by having your pet spayed or neutered."

Wholesale castration of numerous cats and dogs is routinely carried out every day in animal shelters across the country. In fact, in most places, a person cannot adopt impounded pets from such places until they've been surgically fixed for life.

Most veterinarians advise pet owners to have this procedure done on their small animals if they're not going to be used especially for breeding purposes. And organizations such as the ASPCA (American Society for the Prevention of Cruelty to Animals) and individual Humane Society chapters in many cities across the nation vigorously support and encourage such a practice as a means of controlling the pet population.

But this isn't without a controversial side. Some people, myself included, genuinely believe that deliberate castration deprives animals, large or small, of the emotional joys associated with giving birth and parenting. The absence of this wonderful dimension from their lives denies them the social satisfactions that come with such experiences.

Affording Some Measures of Relief

But for countless owners everywhere who've allowed their pets to be spayed or neutered, I offer the following simple suggestions that will afford a measure of relief to them as well as promote rapid wound healing.

Bathe the incision with a solution consisting of a dozen drops of calendula or yucca tincture, ten drops of ionic minerals from the Great Salt Lake, six drops of goldenseal fluid extract, and three to four drops of yarrow extract in one cup of distilled water. Mix thoroughly before using. Tape several cotton swabs together, dip in the solution, and apply to the external incision. Repeat this procedure morning, noon, and night for a few days.

Crush a vitamin C tablet (250 mgs.) and add it to your pet's food. Prick the end of one capsule each of vitamins A (5,000 I.U.), D (100 I.U.), and E (100 I.U.), and squeeze the contents into the food as well. Adding ten drops of liquid Japanese aged-garlic extract to animal chow is also good. All of these nutrients help to promote internal healing and prevent infection from occurring in the area where the surgery has been performed. (Consult the Product Appendix under Holistic Animal Care, Trace Minerals Research, Naturally Vitamins, and Wakunaga of America to obtain the items mentioned here.)

A few veterinarians I know have recommended that pet owners add between several tablespoons of liquid aloe vera to their animals' drinking water as well as rubbing the exterior incision to prevent scar tissue from forming.

STRESS

What Relaxes Animals

Animals get stressed just as people do. Everything from loud noises and bright lights to crowded places and strange locations can make pets jumpy and irritable.

Some of the same things that calm the animals' owners work equally well for them. A nice, gentle massage helps relax tense muscles. So does hand stroking and brushing. Animals seem to like being touched in a loving way when they're under a lot of stress. Finger and hand caressing seems to help their bodies unwind and put them at ease.

Soft music works its own kind of magic. Animal psychologists discovered some years ago that not only does music "soothe the savage beast" within, but it changes the mood and behavior of pets as well. Fear and aggression are replaced by calmness and peace. When soothing sounds are played, inner anxieties disappear. Animals no longer are frustrated but feel a sense of confidence within themselves.

Different botanicals offer relief from stress as well. The preferred herb for a panicky pussy is some warm catnip tea. A soothing tea made from chamomile flowers is just as effective. Tincture of St. John's Wort (six drops to one-half cup water) relaxes a feline or tom. Skullcap herb (one capsule emptied into food and mixed) calms the nervous system. Formulas containing valerian and hops or nutrients such as essential amino acids and B-complex vitamins regulate hyperactivity, aggression, and mood disorders in cats. (See Product Appendix under Holistic Animal Care.)

Animal Therapy Good for People

A great deal of research has been done with the effects of animal companionship on the elderly. The evidence conclusively proves that single seniors who connect with a cat or dog live longer, enjoy life more, and have far fewer health problems as a rule (assuming they're not allergic) than do those who have no pets.

A number of U.S. presidents through the course of history have received their own special benefits from the many different animals they've owned. In a recently published book, *First Dogs: American Presidents and Their Best Friends,* by Roy Rowan and Brooke Janis (Algonquin Books of Chapel Hill: 1997) we find that some famous pooches helped to relieve some of the political stresses attached to the duties of the Oval Office. Franklin D. Roosevelt agonized over events connected with World War II and couldn't sleep well until his wife, Eleanor, bought him a little dog. The President trained Fala to stand on his hind legs whenever the national anthem was being played. The only part Fala failed to muster was a salute with his right paw. But he followed FDR everywhere and provided many hours of wonderful companionship for the president. Roosevelt was able to sleep normally again with his little dog curled up beside him on the bedspread.

The first cat in the White House was brought there by Abraham Lincoln, who took particular pride and comfort in it. The cat was fond of resting in his master's lap, as the president's large hand methodically stroked it while in deep thought or conversation with someone else. In more recent times, the position of First Cat has been occupied by Socks, the pet of Hillary Clinton and her daughter, Chelsea.

But after Chelsea went off to college, her father, President Bill Clinton, decided that he wanted a pet of his own. There soon appeared around the White House compound a feisty little dog given the name of Buddy by the commander-in-chief. This was in recognition of his "beloved" uncle who died in early 1997 and had spent the last 50 years of his life training dogs. Insiders claimed that Clinton has become "less uptight" since acquiring the dog.

Buddy joins other dogs who face-licked their way through American history. In 1952 Dwight Eisenhower was considering several names to run with on the Republican ticket for the vice presidency. Richard M. Nixon's name was proposed, but Ike dismissed it after several aides informed him the man was too "mean looking and ill tempered." Upon hearing this, Nixon went out and promptly got himself a lovable little mutt that he named Checkers. After Eisenhower saw him several times with this dog, he reconsidered and asked Nixon to join him on the ticket. This animal, it seems, made Nixon appear to be more warm and friendly than he really was.

When George Bush was president, both he and his wife obtained a great deal of joy from their companionship with Millie, a lovely black and white springer spaniel. While at the presidential retreat Camp David in Maryland, on some weekends, both he and Barbara would walk and play with the dog. The president was able to forget the burdens of his office for awhile and enjoy life with this adorable and affectionate canine.

As has been shown, pets are good for people's health—even for those residing at 1600 Pennsylvania Avenue in Washington, D.C.

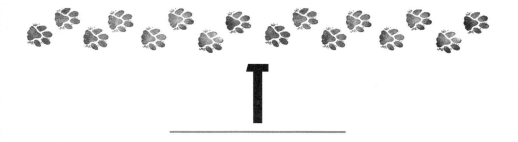

T

TICKS

A Growing National Problem

Once thought to be a problem confined just to animals grazing (cattle and sheep) or traveling (horses and hunting dogs) in primitive wilderness areas, ticks have now become a major problem of many suburban environments. As land developers and contractors have built more expensive homes in or near virgin forests and on open prairies and by coastlines, domestic pets have come in closer contact with these tiny blood-feeding parasites that are closely related to scorpions, spiders, and mites.

Looking for the Problem Can Be Tricky

Diagnosis of a household pet for possible tick parasitism isn't all that easy, considering just how tiny these anthropods are. The skin of the animal should be carefully examined not only by sight but also with a magnifying glass if necessary. One should look for the presence of currently attached ticks or for tick-feeding cavities left by replete ticks as they detach. The average tick will look something like a single piece of black-pepper grain, except that it moves periodically.

Diagnosis of tick-borne diseases has to be made by an animal-care specialist who is well qualified to evaluate the epidemiologic considerations for each disease and look for a previous history of tick parasitism with the pet in question.

Simple Treatments

Ticks should be removed as quickly as possible. This is important in order to limit the time available for possible transmission of harmful neurotoxins or pathogens that they may be carrying. In the past, removal was usually done with a pair of fine-pointed tweezers. But now there is a more reliable way to extract them: a cylindrical, surgical-steel device called a TickPick. (See Product Appendix under Scandinavian Naturals.)

Once the entire body has been taken out, the area should be immediately washed with some soap and water to prevent local inflammation of secondary infection. Some pet owners with whom I've spoken about this problem prefer to give their animals a second skin rinse with a solution of liquid vitamin C. One-half cup of the regular liquid vitamin C is diluted with one-and-a-half cups of water, and the area surrounding where the tick was removed is soaked well with this solution. Ten or so vitamin-C tablets may be crushed and added to one pint of apple-cider vinegar and used in the previously described manner. Cotton balls and cotton swabs come in handy for localizing the treatment.

A unique tick collar (Preventic Collar) for dogs contains amitraz, which acts to prevent attachment of new ticks and to induce ticks already attached to detach. It is available at some pet stores and veterinary clinics. Spraying some tea-tree oil, melaleuca, or eucalyptus oil on the preferred tick-feeding cavities of animals will often prevent their recurrence.

(Consult Lyme Disease for additional data.)

TOOTH TARTAR/TOOTH PROBLEMS

"Sassie, Son of Lassie"

In the latter part of January 1998 I was invited by a local film-casting agency to come on the set of a special commercial then being filmed in Utah. The person who extended the invitation knew I had been diligently working on this pet book for a number of months and thought this particular shooting might be of interest to me.

All I was told was that I would meet "a great Hollywood legend," who was in town doing a commercial for Smith's Food and Drug Centers. The spot would air during the 1998 Nagano Olympics in Japan on KUTV-Channel 2 and remind local viewers of the Winter Olympic Games that Salt Lake City would be hosting in the year 2002.

The star, I found out, was none other than Lassie. That's right, the loyal border collie of film and TV fame. This particular Lassie, I learned from its longtime trainer, Robert Weatherwax, was actually the eighth-generation Lassie. Lassie came into being in a 1943 movie. But it wasn't until the 1950s, 1960s, and 1970s that the dog's popularity greatly mushroomed in three different versions of network TV shows that would all later run in afternoon syndication.

I could sense, as I stood there, looking at the current version, who is seven years old and weighs 93 pounds (the heaviest of all of them to play the part), that I was really viewing a great American icon. Probably more so with today's adults than with today's young children. Those of my generation grew up with this dog and its several different versions.

I watched as his ("Lassie" is always a male dog) trainer quietly brought him out of a nearby trailer that had an imprint of a dog's paw on the door enclosed in a circle instead of the familiar star that is seen on the trailers of actors and actresses. I was later informed that he is nearly always kept in seclusion until needed to keep him calm and focused. Exposure to cast and crew would excite him and probably cause him to "forget his lines[?]."

Weatherwax and an assistant carefully coordinated the dog's interactions with the human actors in the commercial and prompted their canine when it was time to act and react. After several takes of one particular scene, Weatherwax was able to relax a little and remarked to me, "It's kind of funny, but he's at a point now where he's almost too good at it. He's done it all so much he'll give you three takes and then kind of lose his energy for it. He certainly knows what he's doing, though."

Somewhere in the conversation, I dryly cracked, "Here, Sassie! Here, Sassie!" while at the same time snapping my fingers and whistling.

Weatherwax quickly corrected what he deemed to be an inexcusable mistake: "*It's* L-A-S-S-I-E!" he sternly noted, while very carefully spelling out the letters in cold, measured tones. I quickly got the drift, mended my ways, and used the corrected name thereafter, if I hoped to continue our chat under the same pleasant circumstances.

Pearly Whites

Not only is this noble-looking animal one handsome dog that would probably drive every French poodle in the vicinity crazy, but he also has some of the most beautiful teeth and gums I've ever seen in a canine mouth. I asked Weatherwax's assistant, who was on the set with him at the time, what they did to keep this Lassie's dental work so "toothpaste fresh."

For one thing, the dog gets his teeth cleaned on a regular basis just as the trainer and his assistant have done to their own teeth. This dental prophylaxis (as it's routinely called) involves removing accumulated plaque and tarter from the teeth and then cleaning that part (called the periodontal space) where teeth and gums meet. "Lassie sees a veterinary dentist four times a year!" Wow! Golly . . . gee whiz! I thought to myself in bored silence. Tell me something I *don't* know.

The next comment enlivened my interest a bit. Lassie's handlers make sure he gets a regular *flossing* several times a week with ordinary dental floss that many of us are in the habit of using every day. This helps to keep tartar from forming. Another, somewhat novel approach utilized to help prevent calculus buildup as well as to strengthen doggie gums, is letting Lassie chew on rawhide materials as much as he wants to. Old saddles and other discarded leather materials make the finest "doggie chews" imaginable.

What a clever idea, I thought. The many years of accumulated sweat from horses and humans saturated these old leather saddles with a great deal of mineral salts, which, as it turns out, makes for very flavorful chewing. Better that than someone's leg, I suppose.

Lassie also gets a special food mix that consists of at least one part of "certain *fresh* items" that are tough enough for him to chew on but not hard like a brick to break any teeth. I asked my informant what these "certain fresh items" consisted of. He gave me a demure smile and wondered if we couldn't hold that question over for another time. Judging from what some other health-minded pet owners and veterinarians feed their dogs, I surmised these things probably had to be raw vegetables such as carrots, celery, parsnips, and turnips and maybe a few fruits such as apples.

Biscuits to Prevent Gingivitis

If tartar is permitted to build up for very long in an animal's teeth, the gum edges begin to get inflamed. This is easily detected as a puffiness and red line along the gingiva next to the tooth. Gingivitis is the first stage of real periodontal disease. If left untreated, the gums will continue to get more inflamed and infected. The infection becomes worse and extends deeper until it gets to the bone around the root of the tooth. If it erodes too much of the bone, the tooth no longer has enough support and must be taken out to permit the infection to heal and give the pet some relief from the accompanying pain.

It is possible, believe it or not, to prevent or, at the least, slow down such gum erosion with a hard type of biscuit that contains antibacterial herbs known to prevent the occurrence of infection. Suzi Berber of Oakville, Ontario, Canada, developed this type of biscuit that actually works. I thank her for sharing it with readers everywhere. Please note that the inclusion of organic poultry organs is to make this more flavorful and to supply the dog with critical trace elements not found in other foods that will boost its immune strength.

DOGGIE DELIGHTS GOURMET BISCUITS

2 cups cooked chicken giblets (gizzards, hearts, livers)
2 garlic cloves, large
1 tablespoon minced onion
1 tablespoon dried oregano
1 tablespoon cut parsley
1 tablespoon safflower oil
1 whole egg
1 ½ cups stoneground whole-wheat flour
2 tablespoons brewer's yeast (omit if pet has allergies)
1 egg white
Parmesan cheese

(continued)

Place chicken organs in a pot (1½ pounds of giblets make the 2 cups needed for this recipe). Cover with filtered water and boil, then simmer for 2 hours.

Preheat oven to 350 degrees. Combine the whole-wheat flour and brewer's yeast in a bowl. In a Vita-Mix 5000 combine the cooked chicken giblets, garlic, parsley, oregano, safflower oil, and the whole egg. Blend these ingredients for about two minutes or until the mixture forms a paste. (See Product Appendix under Vita-Mix for more information.)

Transfer it to a mixing bowl. Using a rubber spatula or your hands to mix, gradually add the flour-and-yeast mixture to the paste. Add oil to the dough if it is too dry; add flour if it is too wet.

Dust your hands with flour and sprinkle it as well on a board or countertop. Knead the dough a number of times, then leave it for about 15 minutes. Roll out the dough to one-half-inch thickness. This is particularly easy if you roll out the dough on a piece of floured waxed paper. Cut the dough into the desired shapes and sizes you want or else make balls and slightly flatten them with a fork before baking. Bake on a lightly greased cookie sheet at 350 degrees for 15 minutes on each side (total 30 minutes).

Remove the biscuits from the oven and turn it down to 200 degrees. Beat the egg white until soft peaks begin to form. Baste the biscuits with the egg white, then sprinkle the Parmesan cheese over them. Return the biscuits to the oven and bake for an additional 30 minutes. Turn the oven off and permit the biscuits to remain in the oven until they are cool.

Yields more than 50 biscuits. They have an extremely lengthy shelf life when kept refrigerated; they also freeze well.

Herbal Relief for Periodontal Disease

Through the years I've had numerous occasions to use as well as recommend a wonderful herbal combo that always delivers a 1-2-3 knockout punch and leaves periodontal disease kissing canvas every time. It is simple to make, easy to apply, and wonderful in getting the results desired.

Boil one-and-a-half pints of *mineral* water. Or add ten drops of liquid ConcenTrace (see Product Appendix under Trace Minerals

Research) to spring or purified water before boiling it. Set aside and add one teaspoon *each* of the following three herbal *powders:* goldenseal root, myrrh gum, and mullein leaves. Stir in, cover with lid, and steep for 15 minutes. Strain through filter paper and paint this infusion on the teeth and gums with an artist's paintbrush or just flush them using a syringe or turkey baster as Richard Pitcairn, DVM, suggests doing in his book (see Appendix II).

Cat Tartar and What to Do About It

In her book, *The New Natural Cat* (see Appendix II), Broadway singer-turned-pet-groomer Anitra Frazier wrote these words about a common feline problem: "Cats develop tartar on their teeth just as you and I do. And, like you and I, some produce more tartar than others, and some produce tartar that is soft and can be flicked off with a fingernail, while others . . . produce tartar that resembles granite. It amazes me how often I find tartar-covered teeth on the cats I groom."

Bob and Susan Goldstein write the monthly *Love of Animals* newsletter. In their November 1995 issue they offered these practical data, which are passed on with their kind consent.

"Once your cat's teeth are [professionally] cleaned [by a vet], you can keep them that way with a short routine every week. (Use the same technique for dogs.) Just take a square of gauze and wrap it around your finger. Then push your cat's lip up to open the mouth. Put the gauze in the space between the tooth and gum. Rub along each tooth, away from the gum. If your cat cooperates, this will take less than five minutes. Also introduce your cat to raw food, especially crunchy ones like raw carrots. The fiber in them will help clean the teeth."

A cat should also be given some vitamin C (250 mg.) and seaweed (kelp granules) in its food; alternate one of each every other day.

Tweety Bird Solutions For "Poor Toofless Puddytats"

In the Warner Bros. *Looney Toons* that decorated the silver screen throughout the fifties and sixties (and later dominated the Saturday cartoon lineup on television), there was a loveable little character in the form of a small yellow bird named Tweety Pie. Mel Blanc, who gave voice characterizations for most of the cartoon figures, settled on a peculiar style for Tweety Pie. "I tot I taw a puddytat . . . I did! I did tee a puddytat!" became familiar lingo to an entire generation of kids who grew up watching this bird constantly outwit his old feline nemesis Sylvester Pussycat.

In various cartoon settings this hungry cat in search of such a delectable morsel always runs into hapless situations where he suffers from physical indignation, such as having all of his teeth knocked out by one very mean and muscular bulldog that Tweety Pie had sicced onto his attacker. In this still somewhat memorable scene many years later, I seem to recall Sylvester resorting to eating baby food in his toothless state as the cartoon closes.

But, in real life, as Tweety Pie might ask, just what do "poor toofless puddytats eat?" This was found in the Goldsteins' booklet, *Super Foods and Healing Meals for Pets*. Susan wrote how her Yam Puree came about. "This concoction was created out of desperation for a woman who came to me in tears because her cat was missing all its teeth and could not tolerate solid foods, or even canned foods. At the time, organic baby food was not an option. Here's what I came up with. Now it's a regular favorite."

YAM PUREE

4 large sweet potatoes, cooked

2 raw egg yolks

2 tablespoons low-fat plain yogurt

1 teaspoon bee pollen

Bake or steam the yams until soft. Leave the skins on. Blend in a Vita-Mix 5000 at low speed until smooth. Mix in the egg yolks, yogurt, and bee pollen. Serve alone or over natural-base food as a topping. (See Product Appendix under Vita-Mix.)

Cats and Small Dogs (up to 25 lbs.)—½ cup, as meal

Dogs (50 lbs.)—2 cups, as meal

TRAUMA

Flower Power

Bob and Susan Goldstein are nationally recognized authorities on the natural care and correct feeding of household pets. Bob is a VMD (that's the Latin version for DVM from the University of Pennsylvania, from which he received his medical certification) and operates the Northern Skies Veterinary Center in Westport, Connecticut. Susan has an extensive background in animal nutrition and emotional needs. They both are fans of mine, having read several different health titles of mine. And together they edit the monthly newsletter *Love of Animals* (see Appendix II for subscription information). They were good enough to give me a virtual *carte blanche* on whatever I wished to excerpt from any of their written materials.

The following data come from Dr. Bob and Susan's newsletter *Love of Animals* (November 1995 issue).

"We wanted to tell you about a life-saving component of your home pharmacy and first-aid kit. Rescue Remedy is a concentrated liquid consisting of 38 flower preparations. Developed in England by Dr. Edward Bach in the 1930s, preparations made from flowers are known for their emotional and physical healing."

The Secret Power of Flowers

"Bob and I have been working with flower remedies for more than 20 years. Rescue Remedy is the formula we turn to whenever an animal is in physical or emotional distress including being at risk for shock. To give you an idea of its value in our lives, we keep a bottle of Rescue Remedy in the glove compartment of our cars, the kitchen pantry, Bob's travel shaving kit and in my briefcase. In fact, I'm positive that Rescue Remedy played a critical role in reviving our Boxer pup, Jack, last winter after a freak car accident. Jack was hit head on by a car traveling 40 mph during a snow storm. I heard the horrifying impact and saw Jack thrown 30 feet into the air. When I got to him, he was coughing up blood. I thought we were going to lose him.

"Luckily a neighbor came to our aid. Before we made the trip to our family veterinary practice, I wrapped Jack in my ski jacket, pulled out my faithful bottle of Rescue Remedy from the glove compartment and administered two drops on Jack's tongue.

"The short ride to our clinic seemed like an eternity. But, by the time we reached out destination, Jack was beginning to take notice of his surroundings and he even licked my trembling hands. Bob's brother, Marty, treated Jack and he was released the same day in his dad's care. Marty, Bob and I all credit Rescue Remedy for keeping Jack out of shock and supporting him during the emergency. Jack's recovery is just one of many amazing stories we could share with you about Rescue Remedy."

"Thanks, Susan," added Bob. "Marty and I use Rescue Remedy before every surgery, before taking a blood sample from cats and on any animal who's nervous or upset. You can use it much the same way at home. Give it to your cat or dog before going to the veterinarian's office, car rides, bathing, grooming—before any stressful experience. If you are traveling for the Thanksgiving [or Christmas] holiday[s] to be with family or friends, Rescue Remedy provides comfort to your dog or cat while you are preparing to leave and while you are away. Best of all, the flower essences are harmless to the body, unlike tranquilizers!"

The Easiest Way to Comfort Your Animal

"Rescue Remedy comes in a dropper bottle. Simply put two drops on the animal's tongue. If you know a stressful event is coming up, give it to the animal 15 minutes before the event. (You can use it on yourself, too, by putting a couple of drops in water.)

"If your animal is ever in a serious accident, Rescue Remedy can buy you time while you seek medical attention. It is a critical component of your home first-aid kit. Rescue Remedy is available in practically every health-food store in the country.

"While you're out shopping . . . , pick up two bottles of Rescue Remedy—one for your glove compartment and one for your kitchen pantry—before you get engrossed with [other matters]. Show your family and animal sitters [these data] and tell them where they can find the remedy in your home. Once you start using Rescue Remedy, you'll wonder how you ever got along without it."

Another good way of calming an injured or stressed cat or dog is to judiciously employ a little peppermint oil. Keep in mind that this oil is *extremely potent*—a little bit goes a long way. Use a dropper, put five drops over an area two inches in circumference. The easiest way to remember how to do this is to use the points of an imaginary bull's-eye target and compass—one drop goes directly in the center and the other four are dispensed evenly on the outer perimeter in a north-south-east-west direction. Another way is to put an imaginary mathematical plus (+) sign in the middle of this circle and put one drop on each point as well as in the middle. Then very gently rub these into the skin or else place a heat lamp or hot-water bottle over the animal to allow for quicker penetration and more immediate relaxation.

I've also discovered in my own work with numerous animals, household or livestock, that rubbing a few drops of this peppermint oil on certain acupuncture or acupressure points known to induce calmness helps a great deal. These would include ear tips, behind the neck, on the ends of the paws, at the base of the spine or where the tail begins, and on the end of the tail itself.

(See also Stress for other helpful facts.)

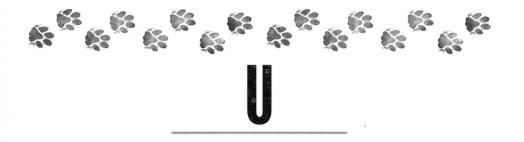

U

UPPER RESPIRATORY INFECTION

A True Kitten's Tail

Here is a true story related to me in my office recently by one of two women who came from the neighboring state of Colorado on health-related business. Alexandria Lord is the vice-president of a large and successful direct-marketing company specializing in the sale of top-quality health products.

"On January 29, 1997, I went to our local Humane Society to select a kitten for adoption. After carefully surveying what they had available, I chose one that was six months old. Little did I know at the time but nearly 80 percent of all the cats confined by this agency eventually die from upper respiratory disease. Within two days my young cat showed all the symptoms of having contracted this very contagious infection. It couldn't smell its food and, therefore, had no inclination to eat.

"I purchased some organic canned cat food and mixed with it the contents of one 500 mg. capsule of MSM or methylsulfonyl-methame (a protein-modifying form of sulfur). I did this with both the morning and evening feedings. In addition to this I emptied *only* half the contents of one capsule of powdered goldenseal root into each can of moist food." (She did this on account of the intense bitterness of the herb.) Within a week's time all manifestations of the infection had disappeared. Imagine the astonishment of my vet, who had examined the kitten before and even prescribed some medication to give it. Within two weeks it had doubled its body weight and its fur coat had changed from scruffy-looking to a nice appearance.

"I named him Aspen Light. In January of this year (1998) I took him back to the vet to get neutered. I kept mixing some of the MSM every day into his food. I'm satisfied to say the healing process has accelerated greatly since the surgery and my cat feels no apparent discomfort." (See Product Appendix under Total Life International for more information.)

Doggone Coughs

Coldlike illnesses can strike animals just as they do their owners. And symptoms can be the same in most instances: runny nose, itchy eyes, sneezing, sore throat, and coughing. Animals, of course, don't have the front-limb dexterity that we do, so they are incapable of blowing their noses or wiping their eyes with tissue paper. And they can't hack very well either to expectorate accumulated mucus from the back of their throats.

That is why they depend so much on humans to help them get over these miserable effects. An effective tea that I've used for treating such problems consists of equal parts (one teaspoon each) of coltsfoot leaves and catnip herb (for cats) or peppermint leaves (for dogs). This mixture is added to one-and-a-half pints of boiling distilled or spring water, lightly stirred several times, covered with a lid, and then set aside to steep for 25 minutes. One-half cup (cats) to one cup (dogs) of strained lukewarm tea is given twice or thrice daily until the conditions clear up. This is one of the best remedies I know of for upper respiratory disorders in household pets.

And don't forget to include 300 to 500 mg. of vitamin C and 100 mg. of vitamin E in their twice-daily feedings to make the immune responses stronger.

Shark Protection

Throughout the Scandinavian countries, many old-timers have been swearing by shark-liver oil for several centuries now. Mariners from

Sweden, Denmark, and Norway usually took an adequate supply of this substance along on their long sea trips to keep them healthy. The shark oil prevented them from contracting lung infections during inclement weather when the air was cold and damp.

Some European veterinarians have been using shark-liver oil in their practices on animals suffering from upper respiratory infections. Since this health-inducing matter is of marine origins, it stands to reason that cats would take to it almost at once. Dogs also seem to like it as well. Small animals (cats and some species of dogs) are given between one to two capsules daily, while larger pets are generally given two to three.

The active substance in shark-liver oil that boosts immune defenses and wards off respiratory infections are alkylglycerols. One has to use care, however, in purchasing a product that contains sufficient amounts of this group of compounds. Unfortunately the public often gets ripped off by brands claiming to have a lot of alkylglycerols, when, in fact, they don't. (See the Product Appendix under Scandinavian Naturals for Alkyrol.)

URINARY TRACT PROBLEMS

Urination Difficulties

Small animals, just as do their human counterparts, frequently suffer from urinary difficulties of some kind. Much of the problem can be traced to the diet. Inflammation of an animal's bladder lining and urethra or the formation of stones is pretty common; cats are usually more susceptible to this than dogs. Symptoms range from repeated urination to bloody urine. In more severe cases, there can be considerable straining or total blockage of the bladder.

Dysuria is the term given to denote painful urination. Pollakiuria is a fancy way of describing smaller discharges of urine more frequently than normal. And incontinence is a polite euphemism for involuntary bladder leakage or when an animal or human can't hold its own urine.

Recipes for Health

An animal with urinary-tract discomforts should be placed on a liquid fast and given no solid foods for several days until the condition shows indications of clearing up. I've devised two recipes for this; they should be made in a Vita-Mix 5000 and then poured into the animal's food dish.

DOGGIE BROTH

1 medium carrot, cut in 1-inch pieces
1 celery stalk, cut in 1-inch pieces (with leaves)
¼ cup barley, cooked
10 drops liquid Kyolic aged-garlic extract*
5 drops liquid ConcenTrace*
1 ½ cups beef broth, boiling

*Consult Product Appendix under Wakunaga of America and Trace Minerals Research respectively.

Add everything to the Vita-Mix 5000 container and secure the lid in place. Run the machine for three minutes. Empty into the dog's food bowl but let it cool a little more, if necessary, before serving.

KITTY BROTH

¼ cup brown rice, cooked
2-inch slice carrot
2-inch piece turnip
2-inch piece celery (with leaves)
1 cup clear fish broth, boiling
5 drops liquid Kyolic aged-garlic extract*
3 drops liquid ConcenTrace*

*Consult Product Appendix under Wakunaga of America and Trace Minerals Research respectively.

(continued)

Proceed with this recipe as with the other: Add the ingredients in the order given *except* for the rice. Run the unit for two minutes. Stop it and add the rice and run for an additional 25 seconds. Let cool, if necessary, and then serve your cat only a small portion of this; refrigerate the rest. An ailing cat should be fed only once a day, and the broth shouldn't be allowed to remain in the dish for longer than an hour. Let the animal get a little more hungry before setting another helping out, so nothing is wasted.

Sarsaparilla tea makes a useful diuretic for difficult urination. Boil a pint of water and add one-and-a-half tablespoons of the herb; cover and simmer for three minutes. Set aside and steep for 15 minutes before straining. Give in place of regular water. When making the tea, *do not* use tap water.

Sometimes a visit to a veterinary clinic becomes necessary if a cat's urethra becomes totally plugged and no more urine can be passed.

Herbal Treatment for Infection

Urinary tract infection in household pets can be resolved with some simple herbal teas. In each instance, use only distilled or purified water. Measure a pint and bring to a boil. Then add the herb in the following particular amounts. Cover with a lid and simmer for only a minute; set aside and steep for ten minutes. Strain and pour into the animal's water dish when cool.

Alfalfa	2 teaspoons
Angelica	1 teaspoon
Artichoke	1 ½ teaspoons
Asparagus	1 tablespoon
Birch	1 ½ teaspoons
Burdock	2 teaspoons
Carrot	2 teaspoons

Celery	1 ½ teaspoons
Chicory	1 tablespoon
Cranberry	2 teaspoons
Currant	2 teaspoons
Dandelion	1 tablespoon
Dill	1 ½ teaspoons
Elder	1 teaspoon
Elm	2 teaspoons
Fennel	2 teaspoons
Garlic	1 teaspoon
Goldenseal	1 teaspoon
Hibiscus	1 teaspoon
Holly	1 teaspoon
Hollyhock	1 ½ teaspoons
Hops	1 teaspoon
Horehound	2 teaspoons
Indian corn	1 tablespoon
Juniper	1 teaspoon
Lavender	1 tablespoon
Lovage	2 teaspoons
Marshmallow	1 tablespoon
Mint	1 tablespoon
Mullein	1 ½ teaspoons
Nettle	1 tablespoon
Parsley	2 teaspoons
Peach	2 teaspoons
Plantain	2 tablespoons

Rosehip	1 ½ tablespoons
Scurvy grass	2 teaspoons
Shepherd's purse	2 teaspoons
Tarragon	2 teaspoons
Wild clover	2 tablespoons
Wild Oregon grape	1 tablespoon
Wild strawberry	2 tablespoons
Witch grass	2 teaspoons

All of these herbs have been successfully used with good success by some pet owners, herbalists, and a few veterinarians for urinary tract problems. Not only have they regulated the volume of urine to be discharged, but they have also corrected internal bleeding. And just about all of them are useful disinfectants against infection of the urinary tract.

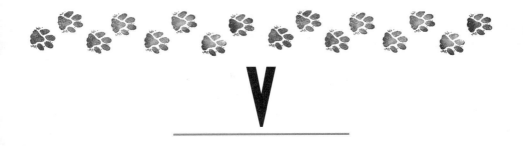

V

VOMITING

Try the Personal Touch

Stella Owens of Jackson, Mississippi, had an 11-year-old black Persian named Satan. For no apparent reason her cat started throwing up when the woman took a part-time job to help pay the bills. Someone told her the problem could be partly emotional, so Stella resorted to the personal touch to cure her pet of its unexplained malady.

She made sure that the food her feline was getting was free of dyes and chemical preservatives. The food was served at room temperature instead of cold. And to prevent Satan from gulping it down so quickly, she spread out the food more thinly over a large ceramic plate; this forced the cat to lap it up instead of grabbing it in big bites.

Stella also helped her animal to relax before meals with a few minutes of gentle massage. She paid special attention to the area around the base of Satan's ears, which is the location of those acupuncture points that aid digestion. She repeated the same rubbing techniques after every feeding, too. She also patted a few drops of a stress-reducing flower-essence mixture on Satan's lips and whiskers as well as adding some to her food.

Besides this, she would pet and stroke her cat more often and allow herself plenty of time before leaving for work to reassure the feline that the daily separations, while necessary, were for only a few hours. This constant reassurance helped considerably, for within a few days all vomiting ceased and never returned. The animal's emotional pain had been alleviated and her mental well-being fully restored.

Herbal Relief

There are certain botanicals that work very well in helping to relieve nausea and prevent vomiting in animals. These are aloe vera, chamomile, peppermint, and slippery elm.

Aloe-vera liquid is readily available in most health-food stores. Give one teaspoon every six hours for cats and small dogs or one tablespoon to a large dog in the same time period. A tea can be made from chamomile and peppermint easily enough: in one pint of boiling water steep one-and-a-half tablespoons of either herb, covered, for 30 minutes. Mix one cup of the strained tea with one-half cup water.

Slippery elm is available in powder, lozenge, or syrup forms. To one cup of hot water add one-quarter teaspoon powdered bark; stir thoroughly before feeding to the nauseous animal. Or crush two lozenges into powder and work into some simple food that is meatless. Or one lozenge (cats and small dogs) can be placed in the mouth morning and evening (double the amount for large-sized pets).

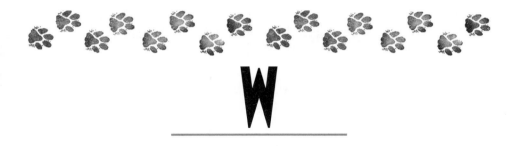

W

WORMS

Intestinal Parasites

Veterinarian Richard H. Pitcairn gives a general explanation regarding worms in his *Complete Guide to Natural Health for Dogs & Cats* (Emmaus, PA: Rodale Press, Inc., 1995; p. 330). He describes them as parasites that take up residency within the intestines of different animals. Younger animals are more prone to getting them than older ones are. However, they usually don't pose much of a problem.

He divides worm-infested animals into three separate categories.

1. Very young animals that acquired them from the mother before or after birth (roundworms).

2. Young or mature animals infested with fleas or those that eat gophers or other wild creatures (tapeworms—carried by fleas and gophers, usually the latter).

3. Mature but run-down animals that are in a toxic state and are susceptible to parasites, both inside (roundworms, hookworms, whipworms, tapeworms) and outside (fleas, lice, ticks).

Five types of parasites will be considered here. One of them affects just the heart (heartworms), while the remaining four (hookworms, roundworms, tapeworms, and whipworms) reside in the intestinal tract. Brief descriptions are provided of each one and helpful information is presented on how to best deal with them using natural substances.

Heartworms: A Pet's Worst Friends

Dirofilaria immitis infection is more frequently seen in dogs, but it isn't that uncommon in cats either. The highest incidence of infection remains in the southeastern Atlantic and Gulf Coast states. Other areas of high moisture content, though, are also susceptible to this problem; such would include the Ohio and Mississippi River basins and Hawaii. Anywhere there is a combination of high humidity and extreme heat will harbor a strong likelihood of heartworm prevalence.

The parasite resides within the heart of a dog or cat; in the former it has been known to reach almost a foot in size, while in the latter it's usually much smaller. Medium- to large-breed dogs that spend a great deal of time outdoors are at the greatest risk. Infection can occur at about any age, but most affected canines are three to eight years old when the disease strikes. Outdoor tom cats are generally more susceptible than indoor males and felines.

The adult worms breed young ones (microfilaria), which enter the bloodstreams of a dog or cat during the summer evenings when the mosquito season is at its peak. When one of these pesky insects bites either pet, it can ingest microfilaria from them and later infect another dog or cat somewhere else. In this new set of hosts the microfilaria evolve through several more stages beneath the skin. From there they enter the bloodstream through veins close by. Once they've reached their new homes in the hearts of another dog or cat, they mature and start having young of their own. Thus, the same vicious cycle is renewed every half a year following the original mosquito bite.

Dr. Pitcairn observes that "a heartworm diagnosis is made when a veterinarian finds microfilaria in the blood" of a dog or cat, "but not necessarily any symptoms of illness." If only a few worms are discovered, it usually doesn't warrant treatment. It generally "requires infestation with a considerable number of worms" before an external determination can be made.

The clinical abnormalities resulting from heartworm infection are quite varied. They usually include exercise intolerance, respiratory signs (such as coughing and quick, shallow breathing), temporary unconsciousness, vomiting (more so in cats), right-sided congestive heart failure (almost exclusive to canines), and sudden death (both).

Help for Heartworms

Different approaches have to be used for treating cats and dogs. Cats respond well to supplemental oxygen. Ask your veterinarian about this. Discuss with him or her the possibility of renting a small oxygen bottle (such as the type used by asthmatic and emphysema sufferers) and periodically administering some of it to your cat throughout the day. Ask your vet for possible suggestions on how this could best be done with minimal discomfort and annoyance to your cat.

Theophylline is another agent that veterinarians employ for cats with heartworms. Generally about 25 milligrams per kilogram of body weight is injected with a gradual release time sustained over a 24-hour period. But there are several herbs containing smaller but adequate amounts of this cousin to caffeine that may be used in place of the intravenous pure drug. These are guarana, yerba mate, and black and green teas. The first two come from South America, and the latter pair are popular in the Orient and throughout the world.

Keep in mind that all of them contain caffeine. The content in guarana ranges from 3 to 7 percent; in mate it is a bit less; and the range for tea is between 1 and 5 percent. During several trips to South America in the past, I've witnessed guarana and mate tea given to household cats suffering from heartworms. The treatments appeared to work, but the cats were sure high-strung on account of the caffeine.

Because of this, I've been prone to recommending black and green teas instead. The usual method of preparation is to pour one cup of boiling water over one level teaspoonful of chopped, dried tea leaves. Put a plate or pie tin on top to retain the heat and let steep for 30 minutes. Strain when cool and give to your cat in place of regular water. It may take some doing before your cat gets around to liking it. But thirst is a powerful persuader and even the most finicky cat is going to drink tea when nothing else is available. The only other option is to force it down the cat's throat. But in doing so, one will certainly face fierce opposition from one's puss. Just keep that in mind if you decide on taking the quick way to get it down your animal.

Sulfur is another good agent for getting rid of heartworms. It works equally well in cats and dogs. Boiled cabbage juice, poured when cool into your animal's empty water dish and left there is of merit but needs to be done for several weeks or longer. You can also utilize garlic several different ways for this. Serving small amounts of minced raw garlic clove in the food of either pet works well. A more convenient way, though, is to add one teaspoonful of liquid Kyolic aged-garlic extract to the animal's food or water. (See Product Appendix under Wakunaga of America for more information.)

Dogs require a little more attention and effort when it comes to dealing with this disease, since it is more aggressive in their species. A canine should be confined to a large cage in order to guarantee it plenty of rest. It is in a dog's nature to roam. But when it is severely distressed with something of this magnitude, its body becomes extremely weak. The diseased heart isn't capable of sustaining much traveling about, so plenty of rest is almost an absolute necessity.

The next thing is to give the canine a good vegetable diuretic. Several come to mind for this that include a carrot/parsley or carrot/wheatgrass juice mix (two-thirds carrot and one-third the other), dandelion root tea, or boiled corn or potato water (minus the vegetables).

An anti-blood-clotting agent such as willow-bark tea or liquid Kyolic aged-garlic extract is efficacious here. So, too, is a good bronchodilator such as peppermint tea if the animal is experiencing difficult breathing patterns.

Sometimes a little common sense needs to be employed when dealing with something as problematic as canine heartworm. A treatment program somewhere in the middle that balances the natural with the drug may occasionally be necessary. Dr. Pitcairn mentions that drugs such as Diethylcarbamazine and Ivermectin, which vets prefer for this sort of thing, are not without their nasty side effects. In spite of his own strong holistic side, he nevertheless told his readers: "I am reluctant . . . to stop the use of heartworm [medications]." His reason is that there is nothing else he knows of that works so well for such a feisty problem.

A Look at Lifestyle

I enjoyed Dr. Pitcairn's section on heartworms because of his sensible approach to things. And also because he includes some original thinking on the matter that had probably never occurred before in the minds of most pet owners. Dr. Pitcairn notes that "there has been . . . an extensive spread of heartworms in dogs all over the United States in the last 30 years." He then lists several factors that contribute to the rapid increases in our mosquito populations.

But in the next paragraph he brings up something worth reciting here and giving some serious reflection to. "Wild animals like coyotes, however, thrive in the very same conditions, even without preventive drugs. The major difference is *lifestyle*—fresh raw foods, plenty of exercise, no drugs and no toxic flea products."

There you have it, a neat and tidy summary of what to do if you want to greatly reduce your pet's risk of ever contracting heartworms. Give your cat or dog a diet that is mostly devoid of commercial food and one that includes few cooked items but mostly "fresh raw foods." And make sure the animal gets plenty of daily exercise. Take it out for walks and romps quite frequently. This keeps the blood circulating throughout the system and can reduce development or spread of heartworms, believe it or not. Finally, keep the animal drug-free and resort to antiflea agents that aren't harmful.

Hooked on Hookworms?

One of the most common and potentially severe parasite problems in newborn pups and kittens (neonates) is hookworm infection. One species, in particular, *Ancylostoma caninum,* sucks far more blood than do other hookworms of dogs and is therefore considered to be the most pathogenic. On the other hand, *Ancylostoma tubae-forme* is the more pathogenic to cats.

The most likely route of transfers into neonates is before birth via the placenta and during feeding periods afterwards. Therefore, the principal focus of treatments should be with the lactating bitches and queens. Suitable herbal anthelmintics that may be safely administered for such a parasite include aloe, carrot, catnip, garlic, onion, papaya, tarragon, white oak, wild plum, and the favorite of many, wormwood (aptly named for the terrific job it does). Some may be given in powders (aloe, tarragon, wild oak, wild plum, wormwood) and mixed in with food, while others may be served separate in liquids (garlic, onion), but included with sweet-tasting juices (carrot, papaya) to mask their obnoxious flavor and odor. Catnip stands alone and can be easily served, at least to cats. But I know of one lady in East Texas who makes a tea from the blossoms of dogwoods when they commence flowering in the spring, and gives this to her pregnant bitch in place of water to prevent hookworm infection in expected neonates.

Square Treatment for Roundworms

As with hookworms, the transmission for this parasite is usually through the bitch or queen, both before and after birth and during lactation. If this condition is suspected, have your vet conduct a microscopic exam of some stool sample. Be sure to inquire if the infestation is light, medium, or heavy and what kind of worms were detected, Dr. Pitcairn recommends.

Noticeable signs for heavier concentration include an enlarged stomach, underweight, diarrhea, or vomiting. When first discharged, roundworms "resemble white spaghetti; several inches long and will often wiggle," Dr. Pitcairn writes.

Teas made from the bark and leaves of ash, birch, walnut, and wood betony are all extremely useful in expelling roundworms from the parent animals. The inclusion of some liquid Kyolic aged-garlic extract in the water of the lactating bitch or queen will carry over into its pups and kittens, which will be just enough to expel whatever roundworms they may have. About 15 drops in two cups of water is adequate for this. (See Product Appendix under Wakunaga of America for additional information.)

Don't Measure Tapeworms

Tapeworms form inside the small intestine in household pets. According to Dr. Pitcairn, each worm has a "head" that remains attached to the intestine as well as numerous egg-filled segments that break off and pass out with the feces when fully matured. These passed segments have the appearance of cream-colored maggots.

You can take my word for it in terms of average size, anywhere from one-quarter to one-half inch in length and save yourself the bother of having to measure them. They are clearly visible in the fresh feces or around the animal's anus. They don't crawl quickly, but "move by forming a sort of 'point' on one end." Once they're dried out, however, they resemble a tiny particle of rice stuck to a hair by the anal area.

The chief problem with chemical worming agents is that while they may kill most of the worm, they often fail to get the head. If it lingers behind, an entirely new body is bound to grow and eventually start passing off segments again.

The best treatment I've ever found for the total removal of such a stubborn and difficult parasite is a combination of pumpkin seeds and garlic. Grind a handful of pumpkin seeds in a small table grinder or Vita-Mix 5000 until reduced to a mealy state. Add a pinch of garlic powder and just enough liquid aged-garlic extract to make a thin paste. Open the mouth of your cat or dog and smear a little of this onto its tongue and hold its jaws shut until the mixture has been swallowed. Or you can be more inventive than this and flavor the paste with a little fresh-chopped catnip or fish oil or beef broth or finely minced raw liver and serve it as an enticing treat to the animal instead.

Either way this remedy is going to work. I guarantee it. You may need to continue this treatment, however, for several weeks until it becomes evident that no more of the worm remains, including the elusive head.

Whip Your Pet into Shape with This Deworming Agent

Whipworms are mostly confined to canines. Typical signs of infestation are: bloody diarrhea, anemia, anal irritation, and bottom dragging.

For pet owners wanting to save some dollars and make their own deworming medicine at home, I've developed an inexpensive but effective formula that's safe for dogs of any size or age. Mix together one tablespoon of rhubarb-root powder with one level teaspoon of ginger-root powder, one-half teaspoon barberry root powder, and just a pinch (about one-eighth teaspoon) of cayenne-pepper powder. (*Note:* Consult the Product Appendix under Pines International to purchase the rhubarb powder. The other powders are available from health-food stores that sell herbs. In fact, the two powdered spices may be obtained from the spice rack of any super-market.)

Divide this powdered mixture into three equal parts and add one part to moist or wet dog food. (This doesn't work too well with dry food.) Use only one part per feeding. Due to the heat intensity of the cayenne, only a very tiny amount should be used. A little practice may be necessary before getting it right.

Another option is to use a commercial herbal blend in easy-to-feed capsules. One that comes to mind was formulated by Lisa Newman of Tucson, Arizona. She included not only my ingredients, but also added cascara sagrada and the seeds of anise and fennel. (Consult the Product Appendix under Holistic Animal Care for additional information.) One capsule per day in moist food is suggested for very young puppies and even kittens. Double this amount may be necessary for older pets.

Some Nutritional Approaches to Worms in General

Effectively ridding your beloved pet of worms isn't as difficult as it may seem. As Dr. Pitcairn so wisely points out: "The idea in treating [intestinal parasites] is to use substances that annoy or irritate the worms and to use them over a long period of time. Eventually the worms will give up and loosen their hold, passing on out."

Certain seeds and nuts do a good job. But they must first be deshelled and ground into fine powder before they can be given to a cat or dog. A Vita-Mix 2000 is extremely handy for this. (See Product Appendix under Vita-Mix Corp. for more information.) Add about one-half teaspoon every day to your pet's meal. Besides getting rid of worms, these items are also healthful for it.

Next in the nutritional arsenal would be wheat-germ oil, but not just any kind. The type I've recommended for many years is animal-strength quality and goes by the name of Rex Wheat Germ Oil. Cats should receive one-half teaspoon daily, while dogs get either one-half teaspoon (up to 50-pound weight) or one full teaspoon (over 50-pound weight), depending on their size. (To order send a check for $65 to Anthropological Research Center, P.O. Box 11471, Salt Lake City, UT 84147.) It also is a wonderful conditioner for the skins and coats of many household pets and larger domestic animals.

Think enzymes for the third item I have in mind. According to Dr. Pitcairn, "the enzymes of many plant foods" such as dates, figs, melons, and papaya, "eat away at the outer coating of [worms]." Dogs prefer dried figs (ground or chopped in a Vita-Mix 2000), while cats seem to like bits of ripe papaya or papaya juice better. If papaya fruit isn't available in your area, then use some papaya tablets (crushed and mixed in with food) from the health-food store.

Implementing a once-a-week fast for your pet is helpful for getting rid of some parasites, especially tapeworms. Without food they tend to weaken, making them more vulnerable to a variety of natural treatments. Permit your pet only a bone and water of a little beef or fish broth and nothing else during a 24- to 36-hour period.

Cleanliness Means No Worms

Finally, the issue of hygiene deserves a few words in conclusion. I've noticed through the years that owners who keep their premises neat and tidy and their pets always clean are never troubled with worms as such. It goes without saying that we usually "sow what we reap." If we invest time and effort into keeping our dwellings spotless and our animals healthy, then their chances of ever incurring worms of any sort are just about zero.

People work hard on things they care about. Giving a pet a little extra attention will yield wonderful dividends down the road when it becomes older. Worms will not be a part of its life, nor yours for that matter (except maybe some two-legged ones periodically).

A Botanical Formula from "Down Under"

Jackie Fitzgerald is an accomplished herbalist from Australia who works a lot with pets and their owners. While she is certainly an enthusiast of homeopathic preparations (just the opposite of what I am), she also uses herbs in their natural state. A formula she shared with me a few years ago has considerable merit in getting rid of intestinal parasites; it is especially useful in treating heartworms in dogs.

AUSTRALIAN HERBAL DEWORMER

5 tablespoons fresh, finely chopped herbs of fairly equal portions or *3 tablespoons of dried or powdered herbs: garlic, ground cayenne pepper, eucalyptus, rosemary, rue or wormwood and ground pumpkin seeds (any of these in equal amounts)*

½ cup oat or wheat bran

½ cup purified or distilled or spring water

2 tablespoons slippery-elm-bark powder (for binding the "pills" together and providing a soothing medium for them to be digested within the canine gut)

Stir the water into the bran and let it set for ten minutes. Add three to four tablespoons of water if using dried herbs. Then add the herbs. Mix in the slippery elm and stir until thickened. If too watery, add more slippery elm. Shape into balls and give directly to the infected animal, storing the remainder in the refrigerator. They will keep for 24 hours if covered.

WOUNDS

Wound Healer Extraordinaire

In a quarter of a century of helping tens of thousands of people and several thousand animals worldwide with a variety of health needs, I've discovered some pretty amazing substances that do incredible things. One of these happens to be pine pitch. It is the natural resin that seeps out from pine trees and collects on the bark. I have recommended it for bed sores in elderly people confined for long periods to their beds or wheelchairs and to older diabetics suffering from leg ulcers. Wherever this substance has been applied, these conditions promptly clear up and the skin becomes like new again.

I have also used pine pitch for treating open wounds and sores in animals. A friend of mine who keeps prize breeding mares brought me to his ranch one time and showed me a horse that had accidentally gashed its hind flank on a barbed-wire fence. I anointed the injury with some pine pitch and left a one-ounce bottle with instructions on how often to continue the application. He called me within three days to say that his mare was "doing just fine."

A simple salve made with 45-percent pine pitch, extra-virgin olive oil from Italy, and a little petroleum jelly works wonders on a small-animal skin condition commonly called "hot spots." This is when chronically inflamed skin develops an unexpected moist eczema. A little bit of the salve is rubbed onto the afflicted areas every day. It usually only takes a couple of days for such "hot spots" to begin disappearing.

A woman from Colorado Springs, Colorado, purchased some of this salve to use on her cocker spaniel named Lulu. The bitch had developed several "hot spots" in the middle of the top part of her back. It made her look funny, her owner reported by phone. She put a little of this ointment on her fingertips and then worked it into the skin by using a circular massage motion. She was happy to see her dog showing considerable improvement by the end of the week.

Another lady, Grace Morgan from Memphis, Tennessee, wrote to tell me how pitch pine saved her Persian cat's right foreleg from being amputated. The feline brushed against some rose bushes in her garden one time and apparently had a thorn deeply imbedded in her flesh unbeknownst to her owner. Weeks passed and one day while Ms. Morgan was grooming her pet, she noticed an ugly and festering sore that had appeared beneath all of the hair on the leg. She promptly took the cat to her veterinarian, who made a small incision. A great deal of purulent matter oozed out, creating an awful smell in the process. Further examination of the leg was made. The doctor informed her that the infection was more extensive than he had realized and recommended amputation.

Grace refused and took her cat home. Daily she poured a tiny amount of pitch pine into the open incision and wrapped it with gauze and tape so her cat couldn't rip the dressing away with her claws or teeth. Surprisingly, the healing came more rapidly than she had expected. The Persian is now doing fine, but obviously has found something else to scratch against beside rose bushes.

Note: I recommend preventing ingestion of pitch pine when using it for external wound healing on large or small animals.

What the Bees Know that We Should Know

In one of my previous books, *Nature's Super Medicines* (Paramus, NJ: Prentice Hall, 1997), I devoted the entire first chapter on "Gifts from the Hive." Nearly an entire page was spent on bee glue, otherwise known as propolis. Bees gather it from the buds of certain trees such as birch and evergreen trees and shrubs. They transport it back to the hive where a special class of wax-worker bees mix it with a little bit of wax flakes secreted from their glands. This then serves as an effective caulking compound to seal any cracks, crevices, or holes found in the hive.

I prefer the extra-thick propolis tincture myself. Not only is it good to soothe raging sore throats, but it also nicely delivers relief to skin situations that may be excruciatingly painful. It works especially well on cracks, fissures, cuts, abrasions, and open sores and wounds. One-half to a full dropper can be used with good results. I've used it around the anal areas of cats and dogs, just below their tails, when such have become raw, inflamed, or terribly sore.

Blanche Waters of Las Vegas, New Mexico, had an American boxer that suffered the sore end of a nasty brawl with another dog. Her pet had one of its ears chewed up pretty badly. She contacted me, and I recommended the extra-thick propolis tincture. She squirted three quarters of a dropper on the mangled ear morning and night. The chewed edges were nicely sealed, and within 48 hours her boxer had regained some of his self-respect, not to mention a healed ear.

(The reader is referred to the Product Appendix under Anthropological Research Center for obtaining the pitch pine by itself or in salve form and the propolis tincture.)

Wound Care with Herbs

In the matter of wound care, antibiotics become paramount when infection threatens to overwhelm the body. But natural substances are by far more preferable than chemical drugs as they usually don't leave side effects and work in harmony with the healing forces of nature. There are three herbs quite noted for their antibiotic activities. Two of them I work with a lot and one I use occasionally but not that often.

Garlic and goldenseal are my herbs of choice for treating existing infections in a human or animal body. They work amazingly well, are easy to find, relatively affordable, and do little harm. The only downside is that they tend to be quite hypoglycemic. For people and pets bothered with diabetes, this comes as great news. But for those with hypoglycemia such an announcement should be taken seriously as they will flatten existing blood-sugar levels, something this class of humans and animals don't need. Interestingly enough, however, Japanese aged-garlic extract (Kyolic) and the fluid extract of goldenseal root don't seem to aggravate existing cases of hypoglycemia as raw garlic or encapsulated goldenseal does.

An average of four capsules of Kyolic garlic or 15 drops of the liquid form or 10 to 15 drops of liquid goldenseal are recommended for small-animal health needs. These may be given internally through food or water or directly applied in the mouth.

Echinacea is okay to use in place of others when hypoglycemia seems apparent. But it isn't something I make habit of using very much. The reason doesn't have to do with any presumed side effects (for it has none that I know of), but rather with its efficacy. Echinacea is one of those herbs that doesn't have very long shelf life. It is particularly sensitive to light and heat. Both factors can quickly diminish the medicinal strength of the herb if it is left exposed to either for long.

Case in point: Some 15 years ago I was in Gainesville, Florida, giving a health lecture. I visited a local health food store with a nice supply of dried herbs in coarsely cut or powdered forms. They were kept inside clear glass, wide-mouthed jars on a shelf facing a large front window. The display was attractive from a marketing perspective, but not very practical from a healing point of view. I scooped a small amount of the echinacea powder into my hand and tasted it with my tongue. I didn't experience that sudden tingling sensation that usually comes when sampling good echinacea. This powder had lost its zap and had the potency of white flour. This immediately suggested an inevitable loss of strength.

   In plain language, the herb had lost its medicinal integrity. And unless consumers are keenly aware of what good echinacea powder should taste like, they would never be the wiser. A proverbial skeleton kept under lock and key in the closets of most herb companies and health-food stores is this: Their echinacea isn't up to par. For this reason above all others do I rely more on garlic and goldenseal, which aren't light or heat sensitive and enjoy incredible shelf life no matter where they're put. (See Product Appendix under Wakunaga of America and Holistic Animal Care for reliable products of guaranteed integrity.

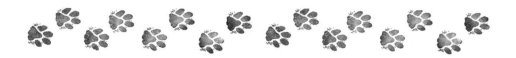

Appendix I: Products

Resources for Specific Products

Anthropological Research Center
P.O. Box 11471
Salt Lake City, UT 84147
801-521-8824

Sells Rex Wheat Germ Oil (1 qt.), $65; Pine Pitch (1 oz.), $45; and Bee Propolis (40% Strength, 1 oz.), $25.

Bio-K-Plus International, Inc.
635 Victoria
Westmount, Quebec
Canada H3B 2V6
514-395-8780/800-593-2465

Sells Bio-K+, a fermented mild combination of *live* Lactobacillus acidophilus and Lactobacillus casei.

Calorad Support Group
6002 West Acoma
Glendale, AZ 85306
602-938-2526

Sells Agrisept, a citrus-derived antibacterial liquid extract and Reformulated Collagen.

Flora Beverage Co., Ltd.
Bay F, 2828—54th Avenue S.E.
Calgary, Alberta
Canada T2C 0A7
403-236-0155

Sells anticancer herbal formulas in liquid form: (Essiac) Essex Botanical Herbal Drink, (Hoxsey) Hoxsiac Herbal Drink, and Mojave Nectar for skin and coat improvements in humans and animals.

Holistic Animal Care
2100 North Wilmot, Suite 109
Tucson, AZ 85712
800-497-5665

Sells quality herbal products for the medical needs of cats and dogs. They feature herbal combinations and fluid extracts. They also carry animal nutrients and one of the best line of pet foods, too.

Indiana Botanic Gardens
P.O. Box 5
Hammond, IN 46325
219-947-4040

Sells over 150 different herbs in these forms: cut, powder, whole, shredded, or granular. They carry many of the hard-to-find herbs such as agrimony, cedar chips, elecampane, galangal, hydrangea, life everlasting, prince's pine, sanicle, stone root, woundwort, and yellow poplar, among others. The company has been in business since 1910 and is probably North America's oldest herb company.

Naturally Vitamins
14851 North Scottsdale Rd.
Scottsdale, AZ 85254
800-899-4499

Sells quality nutritional supplements for human and animal health needs. German technology and attention to details are what make their products so superior.

Nature's Answer
320 Oser Ave.
Hauppauge, NY 11788
800-645-5720 (In NY: 800-439-2324)

Sells low-alcohol and alcohol-free herbal fluid extracts, and herbal creams such as Arnica Herbal Cream. This is the consumer division of Bio-Botanica, a pharmaceutically licensed manufacturer that makes quality herbal extracts for the food and beverage and perfume industries in North America and parts of Europe.

Pines International
P.O. Box 1107
Lawrence, KS 66044
1-800-697-4637/913-841-6016

Sells North America's best organic chlorophyll and vegetable-derived products: Wheat Grass (juice extract and tablets), Barley Grass (juice extract and tablets), Mighty Greens (powder and tablet), Pet Greens (animal chlorophylls), Beet Root (juice extract), and Rhubarb (powder). No one else grows and makes better cereal grass chlorophylls for human and animal nutritional requirements than this company does. It is owned and operated by private farmers in America's heartland, the Midwest.

Purely for Pets
3438 East Lake Road, Suite 14
Palm Harbor, FL 34685
800-426-4256

Andi Brown sells Dream Coat and a number of other pet-care products. Readers may be interested in knowing that both Dr. Richard Pitcairn and Anitra Frazier mention her products in their respective books (see Appendix II). My friend Ron Hamilton of St. Petersburg, Florida, has worked closely with Andi in helping her develop a few of her special products.

Scandinavian Naturals
13 North Seventh Street
Perkasie, PA 18944
215-453-2505

Sells quality health products from Europe for human and animal needs: Alkyrol (shark liver oil), Strix (potent bilberry extract), Original Silica (potent horsetail extract), and TickPick (tick-removal appliance kit). For more than two decades they have been serving Europe, Asia, and North America with these unique items.

Total Life International, Inc.
1355 South 8th Street
Colorado Springs, CO 80906
800-447-4303/719-577-0010

Sells MSM Complete Renewal (a protein-modifying sulfur compound for general well-being) and Cool Whey (a milk substitute made from whey for humans and pets allergic to regular milk).

Trace Minerals Research
1990 West 3300 South
Ogden, UT 84401
800-624-7145

Sells a complete line of ionic minerals harvested from the north end of the Great Salt Lake where the water is the purest. Top-selling products include liquids such as ConcenTrace (a full-strength and total-mineral supplement) and Inland Sea Water, Arth-X Plus, Calcium-Magnesium, and Within-In (promotes healthy skin in people and shiny coats in pets). A full money-back or product-replacement guarantee has been the company's policy since they've been in business. Look nowhere else than here for the mineral needs of yourself or your pets.

Vita-Mix Corporation
8615 Usher Road
Cleveland, OH 44138
800-848-2649

Sells the world's leading juicer-blender, the Vita-Mix 5000. This is the only unit to include all of the fruit and vegetable fiber; no other juicer or blender is capable of doing this. It is so simple to operate even a child can comprehend it. The machine cleans in about 45 seconds or less. The company also sells the Vita-Vac, a special multi-filtered cleaning machine for those suffering from respiratory problems who need a dust- and allergen-free environment in which to live.

Wakunaga of America Co., Ltd.
23501 Madero
Mission Viejo, CA 92691-2744
800-421-2998

Sells the greatest garlic product on the planet, Kyolic aged-garlic extract. It comes in a number of formulations, being expertly combined with a variety of herbs for various health needs. Some of these include Kyo-Ginseng (for sexual rejuvenation), Kyo-Chrome (for blood-sugar management), and Kyo-Dophilus (for improved digestion and food assimilation). I've said it before and I'll say it again: *Nobody* knows as much about garlic manufacturing as the Japanese do. Wakunaga Pharmaceutical Co. virtually wrote the book on what it takes to make a *superior* garlic product.

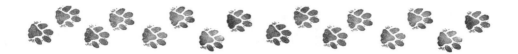

APPENDIX II: BIBLIOGRAPHY

SUGGESTED READING

The following titles may be of general interest or benefit to the owners and doctors of small animals.

Lynn Allison, *How to Talk to Your Cat* (Globe Communications Corp., 1997).

Arline Bleecker, *The Secret Life of Cats* (Globe Communications Corp., 1997).

Dawn M. Boothe, DVM, MS, PhD, *Boothe's Small Animal Formulary,* 4th Ed. (AAHA Press, 1997).

Juliette de Pairacli-Levy, *The Complete Herbal Book for the Dog* (Arco Publishing, Inc., 1970).

Nicholas H. Dodman, BVMS, MRCVA, *The Cat Who Cried for Help: Attitudes, Emotions and the Psychology of Cats* (Bantam Books, 1997).

———, *The Dog Who Loved Too Much* (Bantam Books, 1996).

Bruce Fogle, DVM, *First Aid for Cats: What to Do When Emergencies Happen* (Penguin Books, 1995).

———, *First Aid for Dogs: What to Do When Emergencies Happen* (Penguin Books, 1995).

Anitra Frazier, *The New Natural Cat: A Complete Guide for Finicky Owners* (Penguin/Plume, 1990).

Rosalind Gaskell, BVSc, PhD, MRCUS, *Feline and Canine Infectious Diseases* (Blackwell Science, 1996).

Benjamin L. Hart, DVM, PhD, and Lynnette A. Hart, PhD, *The Perfect Puppy* (W. H. Freeman, 1987).

Ernest H. Hart and Allan H. Hart, BVSc, *The Complete Guide to All Cats* (Charles Scribner's Sons, 1980).

John Heinerman, PhD, *Healing Animals with Herbs* (BiWorld Publishers, 1983).

Francis Hunter, *Homeopathic First-Aid Treatment for Pets* (Thorsons/HarperCollins, 1984).

Bobbie Mammato, DVM, MPH, *Pet First Aid: Cats and Dogs* (Mosby, 1997).

Pat McKay, *Natural Immunity: Why You Should NOT Vaccinate!* (Oscar Publications, 1997).

————, *Reigning Cats & Dogs: Good Nutrition for Healthy Happy Animals* (Oscar Publications, 1997)

Shawn Messonnier, DVM, *Your Kitten's First Year* (Seaside Press, 1997).

Mary and Herb Montgomery, *Your Aging Pet: Make the Senior Years Healthy and Rewarding* (Montgomery Press, 1997).

Richard H. Pitcairn, DVM, PhD, and Susan Hubble Pitcairn, MS, *Dr. Pitcairn's Complete Guide to Natural Health for Dogs & Cats* (Rodale Press, 1995).

Clarice Rutherford, *How to Raise a Puppy You Can Live With,* 2nd Edition (Alpine Publications, Inc., 1992).

School of Veterinary Medicine at the University of California–Davis, *UC Davis Book of Dogs* (HarperCollins, 1995).

Todd R. Tams, DVM (Ed.), *Handbook of Small Animal Gastroenterology* (W. B. Saunders, 1996).

Larry P. Tilley, DVM, and Francis W. K. Smith, Jr., DVM, *The Five Minute Veterinary Consult—Canine and Feline* (Williams & Wilkins, 1996).

Barbara Woodhouse, *No Bad Dogs—The Woodhouse Way* (Summit Books, 1982).

You can acquire any of the preceding titles in one of several different ways. If the book is still in print (and many of them are), you may go to a local bookstore (either privately owned or one of the chains such as Borders or Barnes & Noble) and have a clerk there order it for you. If the book is out of print, you may want to contact the publisher to see if any copies might still be available. To do this you would consult the book sellers' reference guide known as *Books in Print* (Vol. 9)—*Publishers* and look up the particular publisher that way. Or you may consult a bookstore specializing in used and out-of-print volumes and see if one is available for sale. If not, then you may want to have them do what is called "a search" for the particular title with other book dealers in the country. Ordinarily a modest fee is charged for this service, but is certainly worth it if you want the book badly enough.

Some titles may be more difficult to acquire since they were issued by "mom-and-pop" presses or were self-published by the authors. These often take a little longer to find. But persistence pays off.

Subscriptions

There are and have been some very good publications devoted exclusively to small-animal health care and management. A few of them have been mentioned in previous books on cats and dogs. But the inherent risk an author may face for listing them is that one or two may cease publication in the course of time. And readers who may have subscribed to such a magazine or newsletter without knowing this end up receiving nothing and sometimes losing their subscription monies that were paid in advance.

Such was the case in December 1997 when *Natural Pet* closed its operations with the Volume 6, Number 6, issue. It certainly wasn't for lack of advertisements, but was due to a steady erosion of its membership base. In the first several years the magazine sought for and received in-depth articles from knowledgeable people covering a wide array of animal health needs. All of the recommendations made were, of course, strictly along lines of care and feeding in keeping with the magazine's own unique title. But as articles shifted to lighter themes and the remedial solutions became more aligned with the animal pharmaceutical houses and giant pet food companies, readership began heading southward quickly. The same thing happened to *Holistic Animal News* and several other useful publications.

This is why I've purposely confined my subscription suggestions to three current animal publications. I made careful inquiry into their business operations to ensure that they each had a strong subscriber base and would continue to be in print for years to come. Of the three, however, I would definitely have to go with Dr. Bob and Susan Goldstein's *Love of Animals* newsletter. It is by far the most informative and offers practical advice in every issue relative to the care and feeding of dogs and cats. Although a little on the pricy side, it is well worth every dollar spent. You can take my word on that.

I've also included two previous publications that I edited for a while. These contain a lot of herbal information that pet owners should find useful, not only for themselves but also for their animals. These are sold as sets or individually and come as spiral-bound photocopied reprints.

Dr. Bob and Susan Goldstein's *Love of Animals* **newsletter**
Natural Care and Healing for Your Dogs & Cats
P.O. Box 809
Wilton, CT 06897-0809
800-711-2292
Subscription rate is $69 for 12 issues

Cat Fancy
Cat Fancy Magazine
P.O. Box 52864
Boulder, CO 80322-2864
800-365-4421
Subscription rate is $25.97 for 12 issues

Dog Fancy
Dog Fancy Magazine
P.O. Box 53264
Boulder, CO 80328-3264
800-365-4421
Subscription rate is $25.97 for 12 issues

Folk Medicine Journal (Volumes 1–2/1993–1994)
The Herb Report (Volumes 1–4/1981–1985)
Sold as a set for $200 or individually for $100.
The price includes all shipping/handling costs.
Anthropological Research Center
P.O. Box 11471
Salt Lake City, UT 84147
801-521-8824

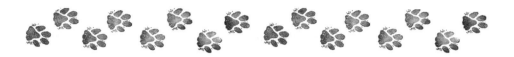

APPENDIX III: SERVICES

INFORMATION SERVICES

Pet owners are always in need of advice when it comes to the health and well-being of their animal companions. The following three resources are information outlets for different needs.

Holistic Veterinarians (in your area)
American Holistic Veterinary Medical Association
2214 Old Emmorton Road
Belair, MD 21015
410-569-0795

(Send a self-addressed, stamped envelope with your inquiry.)

Veterinary Consultations (by telephone or mail)
Robert S. Goldstein, VMD
Northern Skies Veterinary Center
606 Post Road East
Westport, CT 06880
203-222-0260

(Call and leave a brief message with your name, telephone number, date of call, and complete address. You must be willing to receive a *collect call* if you want a short response back. Send a self-addressed, stamped envelope along with any inquiry made by mail.)

Nutritional/Herbal Information (by telephone or mail)
John Heinerman, Ph.D.
Anthropological Research Center
P.O. Box 11471
Salt Lake City, UT 84147
801-521-8824

(There is *no* message answering machine if you call and are unable to get someone. You will have to try again later on several times. On the East Coast, always call
before 10:30 A.M. In the Midwest, call only *before* 9:30 A.M. And on the West Coast,
call no later than 7:30 A.M. If I am unavailable at the time you call, be sure to leave
your name and a telephone number where you may be reached. Speak slowly and
clearly; repeat both name and number and have the message taker repeat them
back to you for accuracy. Be willing to accept a *collect call* from me when I am
able to contact you. If inquiring by mail, always include a self-addressed, stamped
envelope for a reply back.)

An Ode to Animal Devotion

Animals are our love and life;
> They give us rest from toil and strife.
The brush of leg or lick of hand
> Tells us where their affections stand.

"Good dog!" we say in gratitude
> And compliment their fortitude.
"Nice kitty!" is the praise we sing.
> For what our felines seem to bring.

May the animals we revere
> And loyalties that persevere
Never from our memories leave
> When they die and we for them grieve.

—John Heinerman 1/31/98

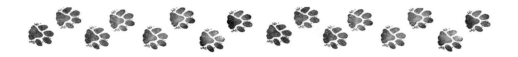

INDEX

C
___

339